MY STRUGGLE TO BE WELL

My Struggle to Be Well

Bipolar Disorder: My Personal Story

AURELIA ROYBAL

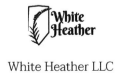

White Heather LLC

First Printing, 2022

2022 Paperback Edition ISBN 979-8-9861157-0-2
2022 E-Book Edition ISBN 979-8-9861157-1-9

Published by White Heather LLC, a New Mexico Limited Liability
Company
white.heather.llc@gmail.com
whiteheathernm.com

Distributed by IngramSpark

Contents

Introduction

This memoir is essentially a personal, thoughtful, and even painful look back over a two-decade long journey of living with bipolar disorder. It contains descriptive aspects of various Mental Health Hospital admissions that I have endured. Actual content from my medical records is included. Basic tips and strategies are scattered throughout.

It is my intention to lend some perspective to this life-shaking, and sometimes, but still too often, life-taking illness. Please come. I invite you to enter my world these past two decades or so, living with bipolar disorder.

One goal of this book is to share and remember as honestly as I can, each episode. Another goal of this book is to offer strategies that might be enough to cause a person to seek diagnosis and treatment, and to encourage full engagement in one's own treatment plan.

Proper diagnosis and treatment, as with any illness, is the key to wellness.

My hope is that you or your loved one can get through this uncertain and frightening time better able to cope. With work, one can break free from the grip of this disorder. Some of the self-care tidbits contained in this book can help almost anyone. When you go to the grocery store shopping, you do not pull everything off the shelves and load it into your cart; you only take what you need. Similarly, with this book, **grab onto those things that may work for you or your loved one, and leave the rest behind, but do grab onto something.**

I take numerous opportunities to give my gratitude throughout this telling. Kindly, be patient with me regarding that. As it is said, and as you will soon see, *"It takes a village to raise a family."*

Dedication

This written work is dedicated to all persons who struggle with a diagnosis (or lack of diagnosis) of bipolar disorder. My heart goes out to persons I have known, or have come to know, who struggle with bipolar disorder. They and their loved ones have much work, and possibly much heartache, ahead of them.

Those that I think of specifically that have somehow affected my life are parents, siblings, cousins, nieces, co-workers, group members, former classmates, friends, fashionistas, technicians, students, nurses, programmers, speech pathologists, certified valuation analysts, IT people, engineers, artists, authors, homemakers, neighbors, church-mates, homeless persons, etc. We come from diverse educational and socioeconomic backgrounds, and a broad range of careers.

What I wish to convey is that regardless of who you are, no one person is guaranteed to be exempt from having this mental illness. I have been touched in some way by so many of these persons, so I express gratitude to each of them. Thank you for all your love, wisdom, patience, courage, prayers, stories, insights, strategies, encouragements, "windshield time", mistakes and blunders, and examples of strength and perseverance. I am deeply grateful.

"Bipolar disorder is not a diagnosis given to a crazy person. It is more like a crazy illness given to a random person."

Claims and Disclaimers

First, let me be clear, I am not an expert on bipolar disorder, nor do I pretend to be. I am simply someone who was diagnosed with bipolar disorder and who is willing to dare to share whatever I can. I hope that it will help even *one* other person, (hopefully more), to better deal with their own challenging circumstance(s).

My views, experiences, and perspectives on these topics will likely be quite different from others. Just like with any illness, you can find a broad spectrum of approaches to care. There are no right or wrong answers to be found here, just personal insights, experiences, and encouragement.

Also, I purposely chose to leave out details like names of persons (such as with family, friends, doctors, therapists), and names of places and locations (such as with hospitals, clinics, cities, states, etc.) in order to focus more on the information being shared and why I am sharing it. I have chosen to leave out names because I don't want to accidentally leave anyone out, and because of how sensitive the nature of this subject is. Instead of getting hung up on the who, when, and where, I wanted to focus on the *what* and *why.* I have also left out large portions of my medical record(s) due to space and personal content.

The information shared spans much elapsed time. As I will explain later, I have a hard time relying on my own memory. So, a good portion of what is shared is a blend of other loved one's memories with my own. It is very possible that dates and situations have gotten confused over time, being that recollection of those episodes relies on persons who were under severe stress. So, if you happen to be a reader who was actively involved in our situation, please bear with me for any errors or omissions as I attempt to tell *some* of what happened.

Additionally, I am a devout Catholic (or at least I make an effort to try to be). Much of my story is woven with threads such as faith, prayer, trust, and hope. Having said that, just as medicine, therapy, respite, and support has helped me, so has my faith.

I do not intend to push my beliefs onto anyone. My intent is solely to share some of the mysterious, scary, and even some of the bizarre aspects of them with you. Some things have happened that "twisted" reality in such a manner that it has challenged my faith. I have had to hold on to it with a mighty tight grip. I simply want to share a raw accounting of what *my* life has been like living with Bipolar 1.

Some Extremely Basic Information about Bipolar Disorder

Bipolar disorder (previously known as manic depression) is a brain disorder, specifically a mood disorder. It causes unpredictable shifts in energy, mood, thought, and activity levels. It is a psychological/psychiatric disorder that lifts and lowers mood unpredictably. It can make the process of dealing with stress and carrying out day to day tasks significantly more challenging. It can often interfere with one's overall ability to function. Bipolar disorder is a mental illness.

Bipolar disorder is typically a diagnosis given by a psychiatrist. Several conditions must be met according to the latest DSM (The Diagnostic & Statistical Manual of Mental Disorders), which is the handbook used by health care professionals as a guide in the diagnosis of mental disorders.

Bipolar disorder is broken into two main types, Bipolar 1 and Bipolar 2. Bipolar 1 has manic episodes (wild or excited mood and energy) that are more intense than those found with Bipolar 2. Bipolar 1 often includes bouts with psychosis (loss of reality).

In either case, energy, mood, and activity can be too high or too low, and can be considered as being in an unacceptable, undesirable, or unmanageable range.

When "too-high", one may experience mania, hypomania (milder than mania) and/or high-anxiety. On the other-hand, if one is "too-low", one may experience depression (mild, moderate or severe), attempts of suicide, fatigue and/or low energy. Whether on the high or low side, one's condition and symptoms will vary from person to person with different degrees of severity.

Cycling between both mania and depression is characteristic of bipolar disorder.

Some individuals have severe complicating issues such as *rapid-cycling* and/or *mixed episodes.* They are worth mentioning, and certainly worth-while researching, if one is so inclined. I will not, however, be going into much detail here on those topics, as I personally, have not had *much* experience with rapid-cycling or mixed episodes.

Seriously speaking, bipolar disorder has the potential to ruin lives. Persons with the disorder are often prone to making poor decisions and often have questionable behavior inside of an episode or mental health crisis. It can be very hard on the individual and on the people who are concerned for their well-being.

Chapter 1

Youth and Early Adulthood

When I started writing this book, I was fifty-two years old, a wife of twenty-five years, and a mother to five young adults, ages eighteen to twenty-five.

I was born the fifth child, the baby girl, with four older brothers and a half-sister. I grew up in a small town along a US Highway in the southwestern United States. My parents were deeply in love with each other, were married, and were growing a beautiful family together. Unfortunately, several very life-changing events happened, and life took a turn for the worse.

From a very young age, there were some profoundly triggering events which caused quite a bit of dysfunction in our family. I will simply say, due to several complicating factors, our parents' marriage ended in divorce. No matter how tough things were at times, we always knew that we loved each other, and just knowing we were loved, helped, I believe, to make us stronger. I made my First Penance and First Holy Communion; in that same year, I started smoking pot.

During the younger years, I was quite a little athlete. I was a tomboy (four older brothers, go figure!) and showed promise in baseball, long-jump, basketball, and a game we called 'baseball throw'. Partially due to family stressors, lack of parental supervision and support, and my own poor choices, I stopped caring much about the good things I had going for me. I cared very little about school, dropped out of sports, and eventually stopped going to catechism (Catholic education classes) and church almost altogether.

Even though I generally used them infrequently, with marijuana and alcohol on board, it is amazing I made it through my teenage years. By age seventeen, my senior year of high school, I entered my first relationship, one I thought would lead to marriage. That year I was chosen for school mascot (I wore an elk costume that my mom had sewn. It had a strange resemblance to Bullwinkle). Somehow, magically, I had also decided to take school a little more seriously. That year, I was voted as Homecoming Queen. It was quite the year!

By the time High School was over, I pretty much stopped partying and was mostly ready to get serious. I had just turned eighteen and had earned a Presidential Scholarship to go to a university about seventy miles away. At summer break from university, I ended up moving in with my boyfriend for Christmas break, after only dating about a year. I had a work-study job as a secretary aide for the Industrial Arts Department and as a disc jockey at our campus radio station. My cousin would call the station to make song requests and remind me *"that blood was thicker than water"* to urge me to play a song from "Air Supply" while I was in the middle of playing "AC/DC". I came to realize much later that the saying just mentioned was so very true.

After my second semester, I chose to study Electronics. Somehow, by the grace of God, I managed to earn an associate degree in Electronics from a community college nearby and was able to obtain a good job as a contract employee at a National Laboratory with a Department of Energy Q-clearance at the age of twenty-one. I worked there doing Data Acquisition, Computer Programming, and System Management.

My relationship, often, was *complicated at best.* We can become addicted to people or things that are not necessarily good for us. Sure, we experienced love, happiness, and good times, and I sincerely loved this person, but relationship issues surrounding alcohol tested me at every turn and at the very core of my being.

After experiencing much sorrow, heartache, and disappointment in my relationship of eight and a half years, I finally had the courage and strength to come out of that roller-coaster relationship around August of 1992. I had bought a townhouse prior, and since then, had been spending time listening to a new stereo, exercising, mountain-biking, fishing, motorcycle riding, four-wheel driving and generally trying to live life as fully as possible. There was a gigantic emptiness though... an emptiness that I would soon discover, only God could fill.

I include this next part of my story because it lends perspective to some of my hills and valleys, and ultimately gives context to a psychiatric term that will be used in my medical records: "religiosity." Religiosity is a comprehensive sociological term used to refer to the involvement, interest, or participation in numerous aspects of religious activity, dedication, and belief.

One evening while watching television, I was channel surfing and came upon a program featuring a nun, who I thought was the cutest nun ever, Mother Angelica. She spoke for a while about various things concerning a relationship with God. I was captivated. She spoke directly to my heart saying, "It doesn't matter what your sins are... Jesus loves you!". It was said with so much love and so much conviction, that I was touched in a way I had never been reached before.

My heart was lifted, and soon, I had the courage to go to Mass again after many, many years. The first time I did, I could barely contain the tears. When the priest elevated the Body & Blood of Christ and said, "This is Jesus, the Passover Lamb... He died to take away the sins of the world." I burst into tears. It was as if there was healing in the chalice. I was barely able to keep my composure. I realized then that I had spent roughly the past twenty years being absent to God. I also realized that, like the famous "Footprints" poem, the reason there was only one set of footprints in the sand was that He had *never* left my side. He had been "*carrying*" me all the while!

Chapter 2

Life before This Diagnosis

By fall of 1992, I had told several people that my focus would be on Church and on attending RCIA (Rite of Christian Initiation for Adults) to receive the Sacrament of Confirmation. I felt that I needed about three years before I would even consider dating.

It seemed as if prayers I was not even praying were being answered. In short order, I met another man, a wonderful man. We were "shot by cupid's arrow" (by his sister, my childhood friend), and began dating around mid-December 1992. For the first time in my young adult life, I felt like a princess (or at very least, I felt respected and cherished like one).

We joined RCIA together. I was yearning to return to Mass and was eager to receive my Sacrament of Confirmation. He wanted to join RCIA because he had been confirmed as a baby and wanted to learn more about his faith.

Before we started dating, though, my mom had come to live with me at the two-bedroom townhouse I had purchased. She had been living or staying with various family members over the couple of years prior. She loved the room I had set up for her and seemed content to be there, although she spent time with friends and family too. My mom was having complications with her Diabetes. She was also having challenges from time-to-time with her "Manic Depression" (the label used previously for a diagnosis of bipolar).

Years later, I would find her journal. On October 9, 1993, my mom's entry in her calendar was: "My daughter told me about her boyfriend's proposal. I cried elation!" We had just gotten word that I was pregnant! My mom was so happy about the news! We made our wedding plans promptly and were married on January 15, 1994. Very hurriedly she began to sew maternity dresses for me. My mom just loved him for me! He was from a genuinely nice, and exceptionally large Catholic family. His parents had raised thirteen children.

When it became necessary, we helped my mom file for Social Security Disability Income and helped her settle into an apartment. She had not lived on her own in years. It was sweet to see her have that sense of dignity and independence. It ended up being very short-lived.

My mom fell ill with what was probably just a stomach flu, but her condition escalated overnight to diabetic ketoacidosis. She was taken to the hospital by ambulance, unconscious, where she remained in a coma for nine days before her organs began to fail. Doctors recommended taking her off of life support, and the family came to agree that this was the best course of action. She lived for maybe a minute or two, but it seemed like a split second. She passed away, surrounded by family, on March 26, 1994, only months into our marriage.

We had our first child in June 1994. We knew we wanted to have at least five or six children, and I wanted to be a stay-at-home mom. So, I gave notice of resignation after our second child's birth. She was born in January of 1996. Our middle child was born in July 1997. Our fourth child was born in January of 1999, and finally the baby, who was born in August of 2000. Without deliberate intention to repeat history, we had five kids in six years— just as my mom had done!

In early 2001, I was a wife and the mother of five beautiful children. I was what someone might call an octopus or a super-mom. Our hands were more than full, juggling the raising of five children under six years in age. One was still nursing, another in diapers, and another was in pull-ups. As with any family, we also had the housework, the yard work, home, and automobile maintenance, and the finances to keep us busy.

We were also managing and operating two four-plex apartments that my husband had bought just prior to our marrying. If that were not enough, we had also immersed ourselves with two home-based multi-level marketing businesses, one after another. What tipped the scales however, was probably the decision to home-school our children.

Back then, my energy level was huge, and my organizational skills were also quite good. I had almost everything in the house organized by color, size, shape, type or in some cases, alphabetically. For instance, each child had been assigned a specific color for several of their belongings such as sippy-cups, blankets, plush toys, toothbrushes and the like. Clothes, closets and drawers were organized by size and owner, toys sorted by shape and/or size were placed in labeled bins and stored meaningfully. Books were shelved by size and type, or by volume or alphabetic order. Items in their rooms were displayed with lots of love and care. Beds were made each day by each child, as able, and in front of their pillows were their favorite stuffed animals and/or dolls.

Looking back after much self-discovery, I can now say I was quite the perfectionist then, having numerous traits and characteristics of one with a hint of OCD (Obsessive-Compulsive Disorder).

A typical day (May 2001) might have unfolded something like this:

1. Nursing first thing (and throughout the day)
2. Spouse off to work
3. Shower/get dressed
4. Breakfast for the kids
5. Bathe and dress kids
6. Start home-schooling
7. Multi-tasking housework (laundry, dishes, vacuuming, tidying)
8. Teaching first grade and kindergarten material for the two oldest kids
9. Playing and reading Pre-k videos and books for the three younger children
10. Lunch
11. Repeat 7 & 8 above in the early afternoon
12. Walk down the street for wiggle time at the park or story time at the library
13. Nap time

14. Finances (time for trying to manage debt, credit cards, accounting, bills,)
15. Field random disruptions from family, friends, and tenants (pleasant or unpleasant)
16. Read and Pray with spiritual material (whenever and *if* ever possible)
17. Kids up from naps
18. Play/occupy time doing something fun
19. Make dinner (~7:30 pm since my husband worked twelve-hour days)
20. Play time for the kids w/Dad
21. Bedtime for kids
22. Shopping and/or tidying up
23. Time with spouse
24. Bedtime (alas!)
25. Rest and Repeat (as a new day (God-willing) follows)

My husband worked four twelve-hour days on, and three twelve-hour days off (and vice-versa the following week). I discovered (through trial and error, tantrums and momentarily hiding or missing children), that it was intensely challenging to shop with all five kids. I usually did the shopping on my husband's days off. Days off were rare because of the apartments. I often shopped at night, while the kids had some play time after dinner, or after they were off to bed. I found shopping to be relaxing after a long day, almost therapeutic. It gave me time to myself, time to think, and time to unwind. I look back at this list now, and just looking at it is exhausting!

As you can well imagine, it took a fine-tuned machine to pull this off on a daily basis. Never mind that this does not reflect or account for sick children, visits, bad weather, etc. It was an exercise in hard work and energy, mixed with lots of determination, love, hope, and prayer. I put prayer last because it generally got dropped by the end of each exhausting day. It's not that I did not feel that prayer was important enough; it was just that my priorities were pretty much out of whack.

On weekends, we visited family or spent quality time with the kids. We went to church on Sundays, and almost never missed Mass. We were in and out of so many Cry Rooms, it was not even funny. The kids had catechism each week, which we also taught and volunteered for.

Our lives revolved around our family and the life we had grown to love. Most of our family must have thought we had gone bonkers, but we just kept on keeping on. What else could we do? Everything we had done up to that point was meant to be an investment in our family. Thank God for family, such as great-aunts and great-uncles. They helped us in countless ways. The kids were well-loved, and we had lots of love and support ourselves.

We took a trip just after the birth of our fourth child in the summer of 1999. My husband was due for a Sabbatical (a seven-week period off from his job at the time), so we planned a once in a lifetime trip. It was to be a road trip, so we purchased a huge twelve passenger van. With a middle row of seats taken out, it fit nine passengers easily. It had a super large cargo space for strollers, playpens, diaper bags, back-packs, luggage, tent, cooler, sleeping bags, toys, books, videos, and enough clothes and essentials to be on the road for just under two months. We had installed a VCR and monitor for playing videos, which would help occupy the kids between wiggle breaks. We were set! We said our good-byes to several worried but loving faces. Without an itinerary or reservation in hand, we headed out on what turned out to be a twenty-six-state adventure.

The trip was amazing! We visited places like Telluride, Colorado, Yellowstone, Mount Rushmore, Devil's Tower, Niagara Falls, and New York City, with breathtaking scenery and fun stops and stays along the way. We enjoyed everything from staying with family, camping, a Catholic Retreat Center, cabins and up to four star accommodations. It was then, and still is now, a memory of memories!

Day to day life was hectic at best. I had no major complaints to speak of, other than that I could not help but feel like I was the main disciplinarian, and that I was the main person keeping things together.

Don't get me wrong. We were **both** doing more than a fair share. We were both working, playing, and sleeping hard. Praying hard was not mentioned, because, in hindsight, outside of Church and good intentions, my prayer life needed work. It seemed that there just was not enough time in the day. I have since learned, *not perfected*, that prayer, devotions, meditation and/or quiet time are all best put first, and helpful if sprinkled throughout the course of the day.

Life was good. At that time, we pictured ourselves being able to vacation each year, and potentially being able to retire rather comfortably at about the age of forty. We had hoped that my husband would be able to retire even younger, so that as the kids grew up he could help with home-school and we could raise our family together.

Fortunately for us, we did not have our dreams and goals set in stone. Although we were young, we knew that God often has an altogether different plan than what we had. Soon, we would be set on an entirely different course, and challenged way beyond what any of us would have probably thought we could handle.

Chapter 3

The Diagnosis of Bipolar 1

(Episode #1)

For several years, since having toddlers about, my husband and I had casually been keeping an eye out on real estate in the hopes of finding a home with land. We often dreamed of being able to raise our kids with the luxury of telling them that they could go out and play, without having to worry about traffic on the street, safety, predators, or the like. After all, that is how we had both been raised.

On Mother's Day, May 13, 2001, life began to resemble a rapid, seemingly out-of-control roller-coaster ride. Stress was huge and my health was poor. I had not even realized that I had gone about four to five days with little food, and hardly any sleep. This was mostly due to my excitement about finding a property that sounded wonderful for our family. I stayed up for hours on end planning and dreaming and staging in my mind how we could pull it off. Suddenly, I found myself full of energy and chock-full of ideas; unbeknownst to me, I was also slowly losing touch with reality.

What I was experiencing was actually psychosis with religious undertones. I had even called a priest, using an emergency number, telling him I was about to experience a miracle. In my mind, far-fetched as it sounds, I thought the Archbishop would possibly be coming to hear my feedback on certain financial issues. More so, I felt a strong sensation that something mysterious or quite miraculous was about to happen.

One thing led to another, until things escalated to the point where someone in my family (either my very frightened husband or my brother) had no choice but to call 911. Paramedics, police and firemen descended on our home. I was still in my pajamas. It seemed that everything good, nice and acceptable was on my right side, and that everything not-so-good, not-so-nice and seemingly unacceptable was happening on my left.

For instance, a seemingly nice, gentle, kind officer spoke to me on my right, while a seemingly pompous, rude, macho and not-so-kind looking one stood with his arms crossed off to my left. After attempting to interview me and getting virtually nowhere things escalated somewhat. I was sedated and restrained. I vividly remember my aunt blessing me, tracing the sign of the cross on my forehead as they rolled me away.

The hospital record states that I was hospitalized for twelve days (May 13th – May 25th). It is mostly a blur, but I will try to recall and share, as best I am able, some aspects of my stay.

It was customary that Behavioral Health admittance was preceded by an emergency room visit. There they ran a panel of lab work to eliminate any physical cause for my condition and rule out any other diagnoses. I have no real recollection of my first visit to the ER other than that nice stuff seemed to be happening on my right, and confrontation and negative things such as needle pokes, etc. kept happening on my left.

Later, however, I do very vaguely remember lying down on a wood bench and a member of the staff trying to ask me questions. This must have been after being transferred from the ER. The hall was dimly lit (likely the middle of the night) and I was still feeling the effects of sedation.

The next morning, I awoke in a stupor. I found myself in a small, padded room, roughly about 5' x 7' in size. It reminded me of a bank vault or a restaurant-sized refrigerator because it had a cold, huge metal door & lock. It took some time to realize, but I was in fact, in a Mental Hospital. The door was left ajar, about 4-5 inches, and a person on staff was sitting outside of the door. It seemed they made notations of my every move.

Later that day, I was assigned a room of my own. It was situated near the staff desk. Being closer to the desk probably made it easier for staff to monitor my mood, energy and activity levels, especially my sleep/wake cycles.

Soon after my arrival, I was placed on several medicines. Some were for anemia; others were for what they found was low thyroid or hypothyroidism. The bulk of the meds, however, were used to treat what I was told was **Bipolar 1 Disorder.** As best I can remember, they told me it would now be necessary to take bipolar meds for what would likely be the rest of my life. I remember expressing loudly: "Bipolar disorder! How can I have bipolar disorder? I haven't been depressed a day in my life!" I told them, "You must be mistaken!" I insisted that there must be something called Unipolar and that it made better sense. Suddenly I was the authority on all things psychiatric.... oh, so incredibly far from it.

The news of being diagnosed with bipolar disorder came as a total shock. My mom and two siblings had been diagnosed similarly prior to this, but the reality of being diagnosed *myself* totally caught me off-guard. There is a big difference between sympathy and empathy. I was unaware of what their follow-up entailed, and lack of first-hand experience and education left me virtually ignorant and poorly prepared for what would follow.

The idea of taking meds seemed foreign to me. I was not one to even take an aspirin, much less a pharmaceutical cock-tail! Not only that, but I was torn at the prospect of having to stop nursing our baby so abruptly; she was only nine months old. My medical records noted I had mastitis and cellulitis. I was treated for breast engorgement and was given Keflex (an antibiotic), and a breast pump. I refused meds and the breast pump to my own detriment, solely because I thought I was fine. I guess I mainly thought that I just needed to return home to my family and to my baby.

That would not happen. Fortunately for us, people around us stepped up in a major way. Support came from every-where. Everyone seemed interested in impacting the kids as minimally as possible. Although it was a major juggling act for my husband and a three ring-circus for the kids, they were well taken care of. This was all made possible by aunts, cousins, neighbors, and family in general. Fortunately, the kids were largely sheltered from the reality of what was going on.

On May 18, 2001, a hearing was held, and the request was granted to "administrate psychotropic medications to the patient as necessary to protect the client from serious harm

until a Treatment Guardian is APPOINTED BY THE COURT"
because of my unwillingness to cooperate.

My mental state was not exactly healthy, and I was hardly
able to comprehend much of this new information. With some
time, I slowly became *slightly* less reluctant to take my meds
on my own in the mental hospital.

Initially, I was extremely elated (quite literally) at the thought
of being there (due to mania). In a very strange way, it reminded
me of a Ritz Carlton, based on a prior stay at one back in the
mid to late 1990's. The hallways had lovely, framed posters of
either nature or inspirational and encouraging quotes and art.
It was not until looking back that I realized that the posters
were framed in Plexiglas, and the mirrors were plastic too.

When room assignments were given, I was thrilled to have
a room of my own. It had a bathtub, which I love, and it felt
special to have the only room with a tub. Even that felt like
my own personal little miracle. Over the course of my adult
faith journey, I have always felt God's presence in some of the
tiniest and tender, yet magnificent ways. It was as if He was
saying: "I AM still here, even now".

There was a male hallway, and a female hallway. The
halls were separated by counters staffed primarily by doctors,
nurses, counselors, social workers, case managers, etc. I did
not yet understand the need for that separation.

At some point, a male patient came into my room, speaking
about some grand plan he had. He tried to seduce me into following this vague plan of his, which I no longer remember. He
then contorted his face in a manner that scared me senseless.

It felt like some sort of evil or wicked entity took over him for that moment. I still cringe inside when I remember it. After the incident, staff was careful to keep us separated; he in his hallway, and me in mine. I became paranoid and scared out of my mind that he would attack me, especially overnight. I could hardly sleep. I was already sleep-deprived, and that did not help my situation at all.

To my best recollection the staff desk was near the "Quiet Room" or padded room. Adjacent to the Quiet Room was a Meds Closet from which meds were distributed, generally three times a day. Both then and now, I couldn't help but think of Nurse Ratched from the 1975 movie, "One Flew Over the Cuckoo's Nest", "*medication time*".

Beyond the staff area was a Community Room that had books, puzzles, board games, and a television and VCR cart, which was brought in for privileged/scheduled viewing sessions. Additionally, there was a small exercise area with some exercise equipment, which I was just thrilled with. If I were not pacing the hall for exercise, I exercised whenever they would let me. I tried to assure them that my pacing was not nervous energy, or what they called manic energy, but just exercise. I was unsuccessful.

Each day began with time for hygiene. I was issued a small shampoo, lotion, soap, toothbrush, and comb. It is not something you think of, but there would not be any shaving either, as I wasn't allowed a razor, and feminine products needed to be requested on an as-needed basis. I was also issued slipper socks for footwear, as patients were not allowed shoestrings for their shoes, and you can probably well imagine why. I wore a hospital-issued gown until my husband was able to bring me some clothing, which seemed to be an eternity, but likely was just a day or so.

Breakfast followed shortly thereafter. The food was out of this world, or so it seemed. Breakfast was usually eggs, pancakes or French toast, yogurt, juices, coffee, tea, fresh fruit (including kiwi and strawberries) and a "veritable plethora" (as a very dear old friend once used to say) of breakfast offerings. Generally held, just following breakfast, was a group of some sort, and there were check-ins with a psychiatrist each morning.

The group included a goal-setting opportunity. I had to fill out a Daily Goal Sheet which had sections such as "Treatment goal for today," "How I intend to achieve this goal," and "Staff assistance I might need to achieve this goal," I had every intention of including portions of the Daily Goal Sheets in this writing. Doing so would have helped to represent mood imbalance and mental instability. I later decided there was far too much there to include.

Lunch was typically an offering of soups and salads and sandwiches, and dinner was, quite honestly, the cherry on top. Dinner had wonderful entrees and splendid desserts. Like I said before, it felt like I was at a five-star hotel. Part of the splendor, in the end, was mostly only the result of having an *elevated mood.*

Due to side-effects of some of the psychotropic drugs, and maybe the contribution of liking the food, I began to put on weight very rapidly. This was a terribly unwelcome guest. During my late high-school/early-college years I had developed habits that led to an eating disorder, bulimia. It took years to finally have the courage to admit this and quite long to be charted officially. Due to numerous med changes over the past eighteen years or so that have now followed, weight gain has been a constant battle. To this day, I see a nutritionist, exercise regularly and must be mindful about my eating habits. I wish I could say that this is all part of my past, but truthfully, I am still haunted by its sting.

Visiting hour at that Mental Hospital was held for every evening; however, I do not remember them well at all. I am told my husband came to visit. He tells me now they even let him visit me in my room. Some friends and family also visited; I have a vague recollection of but a few of these visits/visitors. The visits I wanted most, those that I yearned for, were those I wanted with my children. The children, however, could not come because they were not old enough to visit, much less to understand. Thank God for small favors and for some unanswered prayers.

I was also given phone privileges, for which I was incredibly grateful. However, all too soon, I was abusing those freedoms by making way too many phone calls, and thus had to be restricted. The hospital soon began to feel like a prison, or minimally, like a punishment. I was routinely given various "Behavior Modification Contracts" and was often placed on "time-outs" (their verbiage, not mine).

According to the hospital records that were obtained for me by my aunt, (to whom I am significantly indebted), it was noted that I spent the first day or so in no condition to attend or participate in groups of any kind. Apparently, in those first few days, I spent most of my time manic, restrained (using four-point restraints, a.k.a. straitjackets), and/or sedated (using 5-10 mg Haldol IM and 1-2 mg Cogentin prn (as needed)). It took almost my entire hospitalization to become even slightly cooperative, thus, only gradually becoming even somewhat regulated.

At another point during the early part of my stay, my husband was interviewed and was recorded as saying I had been thinking about wanting to become a nun. When I read this in the record, now in 2019, I laugh slightly, but deep in my heart I have known, somehow, that becoming a nun always tugged a bit on my heart, although I never felt qualified or worthy. Seeing it mentioned in two or more places in the record, it was not a huge revelation, although it was a surprise.

When I was confirmed in the Catholic Church at the age of twenty-seven, the same week as my mother's passing, I wholeheartedly confirmed my faith in God and chose to align with the teachings of the Catholic Church. I had made every effort to live according to those values. I didn't cuss, I hardly drank, I avoided things in my life that I felt were either sinful or could lead one into sinfulness, and I lived my life as good and as pleasing to God as I felt I could. So, when persons in the unit cussed profusely, and/or were having challenges with substance & alcohol abuse in the same ward as me, it made me extremely uncomfortable and quite anxious. After all, I was coming from an environment of ABCs, 123s, and G-Rated movies.

At some point, there was a male patient who was choosing the video we would watch that evening. He went to a specific cabinet where all the videos were labeled "ADULT", which completely unraveled me. I said, "No way! We shouldn't all have to watch 'ADULT' movies just because *he* likes them!" They then had to explain to me that most of the movies were rated PG-13 or R, and that they were labeled that way simply to distinguish those that were labeled "ADULT" as the ones stored in the adult wing, from those labeled "ADOLESCENT" for those stored in the adolescent wing. Looking back on this, it's funny, but I still prefer rated PG movies.

In the upcoming paragraphs, I have taken summaries or excerpts from my Mental Health Records. Keep in mind that these are but a page or two taken from inches upon inches from each episode. This will hopefully give you a tiny glimpse of my mental state upon each admittance, and any improvement, if at all, upon each discharge. Each episode/hospitalization record has been entered in block text.

The Discharge Summary of my first hospitalization contained information such as:

ADMISSION DATE: 5/13/01

DISCHARGE DATE: 5/25/01

REASON FOR ADMISSION: This 34-year-old female had become rapidly and severely manic during the week prior to admission. She had slept very little during the five days prior to admission. She also developed pressured speech, physical hyperactivity. Had flight of ideas and difficulty with concentration. She also began to voice paranoid and grandiose thoughts. Her condition would go to the point where she was unable to care for herself and her five young children.

Also, this reportedly was her first clear manic episode, though does have a family history of bipolar disorder.

MENTAL STATUS EXAMINATION: At the admission, the patient's speech was quite rapid. She also had racing thoughts.

She had excessive religious ideation. She stated that she had "been through a miracle". She reported her mood as "great" and also that she had been thinking about "everything" over the week and had developed many important insights that were "very powerful for me". At admission, the patient appeared quite manic with pressured speech and loose association. She also had grandiosity and was minimally cooperative with the interview due to her manic and agitated state.

HOSPITAL COURSE: Patient continued to be quite manic during the early part of this admission. She initially refused any medication. At times she was agitated, even assaultive. She was restrained twice. Had to be given Haldol injections on two occasions.

She gradually accepted the need for medication. Was started on Zyprexa initially 20 mg at h.s. Still had difficulty complying with the Zyprexa. Had to write a flexible schedule, wrote for Zyprexa 5 mg in the morning, 5 mg at 1700, 10 mg at h.s. Also wrote for 5mg p.o. up to twice a day p.r.n. as needed as patient would occasionally refuse her dose though later request the dose. During the mid-part of her stay, she did comply more with taking the Zyprexa, also on 5/22/01 went ahead with a Depakote trial, though the patient developed a rash and it had to be discontinued. She continued to have difficulty with sleep throughout this stay. It did also help for her to take an additional Haldol 5 mg at h.s..

By discharge, the patient, though she remained hypomanic, requested discharge. Her husband also wanted to see if she could manage things out of the hospital. Patient agreed to take her medication. They also had made arrangements for her to stay at her brother [in-law]'s home so that she would not have to go to her home and right away deal with the demands of running her household.

PROGNOSIS: Guarded at discharge, largely due to patient's continued denial of the severity of her illness.

DISCHARGE DIAGNOSIS: DSM-IV

Axis I: Bipolar I disorder, current episode manic with psychotic features.

Axis II: No diagnosis.

Axis III: Patient has five young children, the youngest being nine months of age. Had breast engorgement at admission with impending mastitis.

Axis IV: Psycho-social stressors – actually pretty mild. Patient is in good health. Has a good marriage.

Axis V: GAF rated at 22 on admission and estimated to be 70 as the highest level during the last year.

A side note worth mentioning is that if you don't know what a GAF is, it is the Global Assessment of Functioning tool or chart that can be referenced to evaluate or "get a feel" for the rating or scale used above under Axis V.

I don't remember much detail about leaving the hospital, other than I thought I'd need to do a lot of laundry when I'd get home. I figured I would likely come home to a house turned upside-down, but mostly I was deeply embarrassed, exhausted, and overwhelmed by the enormity of it all. My husband became hungry for knowledge. I, on the other hand, was not a reader by nature, and was content to follow the school of hard knocks. At this time, there was hardly anything written about bipolar. My husband bought a thick, fairly exhaustive book on the chemistry and condition of the brain and on how medication works/reacts with it.

Realistically, though, neither my husband nor I were prepared for the follow-up that would be necessary. He remembers being sent home with a boatload of verbal and written communication—paperwork galore. This included several prescriptions that needed filling, a follow-up therapy appointment, a follow-up psychiatry appointment, and basic information such as release notes and discharge forms.

Both my husband and I seemed to agree that it was too much to do, not enough time to do it, and how could we pull it all off anyhow? I had pretty much convinced my husband I did not need it, and that they were just going to have me re-hash my past, and get into my head, put things in my head, and maybe even make me believe I was worse off than what I really was. Ok, so I also had trust issues.

Prior to this time, as a teenager and young adult, I remember regarding therapy as being something for celebrities, and psychiatry as basically being bogus. I thought of psychiatrists as "shrinks", and both therapists and psychiatrists as being reserved for either the wealthy or for the weak, and otherwise used for people who were in desperate need, such as with persons with extremely severe mental problems.

Now, looking back, I am eternally grateful to my providers. Stigma almost prevented me from getting the great care I have gotten over the years.

Something I have learned, primarily through individual therapy, is how to better handle the stress common to everyday life as we know it. Two heads are often better than one, and at least as far as my experience is concerned, it is better to seek out and get professional help than to put unnecessary strain on any of my relationships.

Also, avoiding episodes, at almost any cost, has been better than having to bounce back from even one. Each episode has a cost: a toll on one's body, on one's mind, and on one's soul. There has also been a huge financial toll.

The financial toll I speak of is mainly the cost of obtaining the care I so desperately needed (individual therapy, psychiatry, medications, etc.). These had become such a financial burden for us (the cost of meeting deductibles, co-pays, out-of-pocket expenses, etc.). The hospital admittance/stay alone was a chunk of money.

It would not be until further down the road that I would be awarded SSDI (Social Security Disability Income) and Medicare. I could then use my husband's insurance as primary and Medicare as secondary. Finally, with those in place, we were better able to afford those very necessary maintenance costs.

Chapter 4

Five Weeks Later, Still Manic

(Episode #2)

After the first episode, we were left dumbfounded and completely derailed. Now, my husband recognizes he was caught by surprise, and we both feel that we both had a profound case of denial. I do not recall following-up with any kind of discharge plan. We were extremely overwhelmed and were just doing what we could to get by. As you can imagine, just trying to fall back into the same routine was hard enough! Laundry was piled up, there were bills to pay, mail to catch up with, and children to tend to, and that's just the beginning.

So, as you could probably guess, my second manic episode was probably mostly due to lack of proper follow-up regarding taking meds as prescribed. I filled the prescriptions, tried, and failed. I made a decent effort to comply, but found it all too complicated, expensive, new, and troublesome. My mind soon told me that I would be better off "natural" then on all the medications. I highly disliked taking them, especially because of side-effects like foggy-brain, dry mouth, etc. Somehow in my heart, I believed that I would soon be back to normal. This was outrageously short-lived and highly inaccurate.

I bounced back into the ER and Mental Hospital, but remember little outside of what hospital records have afforded me. They say that I was admitted on June 21, 2001 and released only five days later, on June 26, 2001. As had happened during the previous hospitalization, I was there for round two of "Bipolar 1 Disorder, manic, with psychotic features."

My husband, all the while, was using babysitters and family in the least chaotic way he could manage. The demands of trying to keep his job, meetings with various staff at the hospital, visiting hours, communicating with both sides of the family and friends, taking care of kids and tending to normal household responsibilities, etc., kept him exhausted. Before all this happened, we were both completely spent at the end of each day. Now, there was mainly only one person handling the entire, larger load. He could not have done it alone! Again, enormous thanks to all the people involved in keeping our family together.

He has since said that he was challenged by the fact that this was not going to be a temporary situation, but a life-changing event. We were both thrown by how little we knew about this illness, especially since it was in my family. My husband seems to recall that I was triggered by the poor health and hospitalization of his mother, prior to her becoming terminally ill. Once he reminded me of that, I was able to recall the enormity of the impact it had on me.

I remember packing a suitcase to go visit his mother in the hospital in our neighboring city. I packed numerous items suitable for a chapel. I also remember calling my aunt who was one of our main supports at that time. I told her that we needed to go to the hospital and that we needed her to come and watch the kids. She arrived in nearly no time at all.

Upon leaving the house for the hospital, I suddenly found it necessary to place a 911 call to say that my aunt needed help with the kids!?!?! Indeed, probably only a mentally ill person would do such a thing. That underscores, for me, the idea that many mentally ill persons might have no real personal awareness of being altered or of "being off". I certainly did not. Bipolar disorder often interferes with one's overall ability to function, especially in the middle of a crisis or an episode or both.

The police arrived at our home in less than 10 minutes. My aunt now says that there was a knock on the door and that two officers who arrived explained that they needed to conduct a wellness check of the children due to my 911 call. Fortunately, she was able to satisfy the officers with the interview and the search of the house, upon which time they departed.

We successfully visited my husband's mother in the hospital, but I hardly remember the visit. I vaguely remember seeing various members of his large family. Afterwards, I remember going to the gift shop and becoming compelled to purchase about twenty to twenty-five greeting cards off the rotating racks. It seemed that each one mysteriously seemed to have a personal message that was applicable to almost any of several of the relationships I had. I must have dropped at least $100 - $125 right then and there, just on cards. This is a tiny example of hypomania, and a relatively small exercise in poor judgment. His sister came out to the van to check on me; she was likely suspicious of my strange behavior.

It has taken years, several hospitalizations in fact, for me to learn what hypomania and mania are, how they feel, and how to distinguish between them. To this day, even with extreme diligence, it is hard for me to distinguish the difference. It's a mighty fine line crossing over from one to the other, and likely, it is probably different from one person to the next.

The drive back home was about a seventy-mile drive, and the wind returning home seemed treacherous at best. I was experiencing extreme discomfort and anxiety. My husband was trying to convince me that the conditions were not really that bad, but I remember it as being dangerously risky. We arrived without incident, but I was completely frazzled.

My aunt remembers packing up the kids and taking the children to her home. I do not quite recall if it was hours, days, or weeks later (likely hours), but this was the rough transition from hypomania into mania for this second episode. I liken mania to climbing a tree. You do not realize how high you have climbed until you are either scared or exhilarated, and then you have to make your way back safely to the ground.

Here we would go again, whenever it was. The 911 scene all over again. Units from both fire and police departments responded, as did the ambulance; suddenly they were all in front of our house. I packed and insisted on a few "essentials", including a set of car & house keys with a remote, which turned up lost once I was transported to the ER and the Mental Hospital. The ambulance ride, once again, was heart-pounding and anxiety-producing. The sound of the motor and the rumble and feeling in my chest must have increased my sense of fear. I could sense every stop, every speed bump, every acceleration. I could feel the ride as if I had super hyper-sensitivity. Each ambulance ride felt like I was headed toward death due to panic/anxiety.

The Discharge Summary of my second hospitalization contained information such as:

ADMISSION DATE: 6/21/01

DISCHARGE DATE: 6/26/01

REASON FOR ADMISSION: Patient admitted as she was in acute manic state with psychotic features.

Patient had been admitted one month prior on 5/13/01. Patient then was in a manic state. Patient then was uncooperative with treatment and would not comply with taking medication.... It was thought that she did not continue her medication and she had a progression again into extreme manic behavior. At admission her speech was very rapid and pressured. She had some flight of ideas with some paranoid thoughts.

MENTAL STATUS EXAMINATION: At admission this 34-year-old female appeared extremely manic. Her speech was very fast. She also had flight of ideas. She also voiced paranoid ideation. She was very intrusive. Physically hyperactive and walked very fast. Had a labile mood which could change from euphoric to irritable. At times her thought processes would approach that of a word salad. She also expressed paranoid ideation. She denied any suicidal or homicidal ideation. Patient could not cooperate with testing of cognition, though at the last admission, patient had good recent and remote memory, though has very poor insight and is practicing poor judgement in terms of caring for herself and actually also for her young children.

HOSPITAL COURSE: Patient again initially refused to take medication. Asked to be discharged. Was considering a discharge. Discussed this with her husband. Her husband came to the unit. When her husband came to the unit the patient's behavior escalated out of control. She tried to elope. She became physically aggressive with staff. Had to be restrained. Then was administered Haldol 5 mg IM with Cogentin 2 mg. Patient did become calmer. Patient was placed on a 5 day hold. Started Zyprexa at 5 mg p.o. q.i.d. Patient began to take the medication and she herself actually preferred the q.i.d. schedule.

On 6/23/01 she remained paranoid though had some decrease of pressured speech. By 6/26/01 she was much calmer, had no pressured speech. Had been sleeping well the last two nights and voiced no paranoid ideation.

Patient then discharged as she requested a discharge on 6/26/01. Patient also agreed that she would continue with outpatient treatment and she made this agreement very importantly also with her husband.

PROGNOSIS: Currently remains guarded due to history of noncompliance.

DISCHARGE DIAGNOSIS: DSM-IV

Axis I: Bipolar I disorder, most recent episode manic with psychotic features

Axis II: Deferred.

Axis III: No Diagnosis.

Axis IV: Psychosocial stressors – moderate. Especially that of severe recent mania with noncompliance with treatment.

Axis V: GAF rated at 48 at the time of admission, estimated to be 65 as the highest level during the last year.

This may have been the episode where I could swear that I
had been groped in the ambulance. Even medicated, there is a
certain sense of awareness, especially when manic and hyper-
aware. Sedating meds, however, made my ability to stay alert
and focused less keen.

Also, according to notes made in charts, this admittance was
awful to say the least. I had flight of ideas, pressured speech,
paranoid thoughts, delusions, etc. Even though I imagined that
I was good at making myself "seem" better than I was, they
mostly saw right past any attempt(s) at manipulation. Truth be
told, I was quite sick, and I was out of control.

From the records, a telephone conversation was noted to
have been about my relentless "urging" for premature discharge. The conversation was documented, and the content
was mainly about trying to convince my husband to convince
me not to keep pressuring a discharge, because if they let me
go AMA (against medical advice), the bill would be rejected by
insurance and billed to us. This certainly was not the start of
my husband's worries and stress; he already had a heavy load.
It was, however, the beginning of the weight or burden of additional financial worries. They urged him to convince/influence
me to stop.

I wish now that I could have had the wherewithal to have
handled myself differently. So much so, that I now dedicate
myself to my wellness faithfully. Information about various
approaches one could take, that for me, have been a benefit

to my overall wellness, is shared in Chapter 11 which is titled "Insights, Tips & Strategies".

Chapter 5

The Aftermath of Mania: Depression

(Episode #3)

Very shortly after discharge from the second episode, a marketing group selling time-shares set up shop in an outlet mall near the property we were looking to buy. As you have probably guessed, we bought a time-share. Over the years, the purchase has been a thorn in our side, costing between $15k and $20k initially, plus yearly maintenance fees. We have hardly been able to use it due to time and money. We have been unsuccessful at selling it. Our hope is that someday we will be able to use it enough that we do not consider it a total loss or offer it to someone who can afford the maintenance fees. Either way, we use it minimally, but are stuck with it for now.

In any case, during the time between Episodes two and three, we finally bought our home in the country nestled between two cities! It was close enough for my husband to commute to work and was a wonderful home and would *become* well-suited to our family, *with some work*. Don't get me wrong

—the home was lovely in the condition it was in, but in order to accommodate *our* whole family well, it was going to need an addition and/or remodeling... preferably handled well *before* moving in.

I was hypo-manic/manic, however, and did not realize it. What I remember is that the name of the street where the house was located was Rose, and that it had roses planted out-side. It made me think of the Blessed Virgin Mary and seemed as if it were some sort of a sign. Everything *seemed* doable, *seemed* practical, and *felt* level- headed. The complicating factor was that I had the confidence and surety of hypomania/mania. This often makes things seem great and fantastic, but in actual reality they are not nearly as grand. It is as though you are seeing through rose-colored glasses, and that was likely the reason why everything seemed and felt fine, even though it was not.

In hindsight, the last thing you want to have on your plate while manic is the ability to negotiate or purchase anything of much value, specifically not high-dollar investments like real property.

As I remember it, the house was essentially a two bedroom with a double garage on approximately three acres. With lots of help from friends and family, and probably lots of hope and prayer (and doubt), we moved in! I don't remember if it hit me that very day, or if the reality of being squeezed into that space hit me overnight, but within a couple of days I had shut down and was begging, needing to go home. I was desperate and quite literally a mess. My husband tells me that my sister-in-law came and took me to her home. I don't remember this whatsoever. I was not in a good state at all. I now know the condition was extreme anxiety, followed by deep regret, then advancing to moderate, and then to severe depression.

My husband had no viable option other than to move us back. To everyone else, it must have seemed like a severe case of "the tail wagging the dog", and in all truth it was, but the tail was not me and the dog was not my husband. *The tail was bipolar disorder, and the dog was everybody/everything in its path.*

Fortunately, we had not yet sold the old house. *Unfortunately*, we had to pretty much forfeit our $20,000.00 down payment, but we were able to sell it to a family member. It seems safe to say it has turned out to be a win-win situation.

This is where my big dilemma comes in. I have decided to share something in this book that has been practically paralyzing for me, as far as writing is concerned. It is something that has been greatly troubling for me since I first read it, and it still makes me shudder whenever I think of it.

In the summer of 2001, our family nearly mirrored the situation of a family in Texas. The similarities are incredibly eerie, horrific, and haunting. A mother with postpartum psychosis drowned all five of her own children. Her children were similar in age to ours, were home-schooled, and it happened within just a few weeks of my second and third episodes. This made national, maybe even international news.

At that time, this information absolutely heightened concern from friends and family over my well-being and the safety of our children. My husband told me that he had to pull off to the side of the road when he heard that awful news... quite literally, he found himself shaking. I myself have no memory of it, and so whenever I had read that I had *both suicidal and homicidal ideation* in my medical record, it hit me like a ton of bricks. It affected me like any earth-shattering news would. It made me uneasy, queasy and sick inside. I was heartbroken.

It is difficult to admit, much less accept, that I could have ever been near any thoughts such as those, not in my right mind, anyhow. It tears me up just thinking about it.

As you could well imagine, it not only felt important, but also necessary to tell this to my kids after this discovery. I did not want them to discover it whenever, or if ever, they would read this book, without first talking to them. I also wanted to be sure that they did not mind me writing about it. Mainly, I chose to talk to them because I love and respect each of them, and because it was the truth. Some truths are harder to own than we realize.

The Discharge Summary of my third hospitalization contained information such as:

ADMISSION DATE: 7/22/01

DISCHARGE DATE: 7/31/01

REASON FOR ADMISSION: Patient was admitted in order to evaluate dangerousness, treat depression and Bipolar illness intensely as an impatient due to failure of outpatient treatment.

PROVISIONAL DIAGNOSIS: Affective disorder, Bipolar, depressed, with suicidal and homicidal ideation.

HISTORY OF ILLNESS: Patient was admitted on referral from Emergency Room, where patient presented complaining of suicidal and homicidal ideation. This was the third psychiatric admission in the past four months for this 34-year-old married female mother of five, who reported feelings of guilt and being overwhelmed by recent move to a new home in the country which did not work out, and patient insisted returning to the old home, and in the process the family lost $20,000 on a real estate contract. The patient complained that her home is now in disarray with boxes, and she has had to arrange for her two oldest children to live with an aunt out of state.

MENTAL STATUS EXAMINATION: Examination revealed a well-developed, well-nourished female, appearing approximately her stated age, who is alert and oriented in all spheres. Mood was described as sad and anxious, and affect was appropriate to mood and depressed. Patient admitted to suicidal and homicidal ideation and denied intent. Thought was fairly focused, some overinclusive detail. Speech was clear. There was no evidence of current organized delusions or misperceptions. Recent and remote memory appeared intact, as was registration and recall. Intellectual functioning appeared average. Insight and judgment appeared fair.

HOSPITAL COURSE AND TREATMENT: Patient was admitted to the Adult Treatment Unit, where she remained throughout her hospital stay. She was treated with daily individual and group psychotherapy, and received psychotropic medications consisting of Zyprexa 15 mg q h.s., Remeron 15 mg q h.s., and Zyprexa was decreased to 10 mg q h.s. and Remeron increased to 30 mg q h.s. Patient received lorazepam 0.25 mg b.i.d. and q 4 hours p.r.n., increased to 0.5 mg b.i.d. Patient participated actively in the group therapies and talked about her distressing situation. Admitted feeling discouraged and feelings of hopelessness. Patient experienced significant drowsiness and sleeping much of the day, and when awake, tended to worry about her situation in the future. Reported feeling numb and having feeling about her children. She tended to be reclusive, but gradually became more interactive and participated in group therapies. Patient admitted to having difficulty relating to peers in group therapies who were involved with drug use and used foul language. Patient reported guilt feelings about loss of money and her two children having to move to Texas. She reported home schooling her children in recent years. Did report having a [sibling] with Bipolar illness.

On 7/30 patient reported feeling improved in mood, decrease in anxiety and worry, and able to redirect her attention and focus on days' tasks with more positive outlook. She complained of feeling bored in the hospital and wanting to go home and get on with tasks of organizing her house. Reported having good visit with her husband and family. Patient admitted being anxious about going home but looked forward to same. Claimed to be sleeping and eating well. Improved concentration and energy. Reported planning to follow up with her new doctor in one week.

PROGNOSIS: Guarded, in view of recurrent nature of illness.

CONDITION ON DISCHARGE: Improved, relief of suicidal/ homicidal ideation, trend of stabilization of mood and affect.

FINAL DIAGNOSIS:

Axis I.   Affective disorder, Bipolar, depressed, with suicidal ideation.

Axis II.   Deferred.

Axis III.   None of current attention.

Axis IV. Code 3 – financial distress, multiple moves.

Axis V. GAF on admission 35. Highest level past year 65.

DISPOSITION: Patient is discharged to her own recognizance.

Upon going home after the third episode, my husband realized I would be unable to continue home-schooling, and that some major changes needed to be made. Truth be told, we were barely keeping things together. The kids were being juggled around between babysitters, friends and family. Our lives and our home had come to resemble utter chaos.

We sent our two oldest children to live out of state with my aunt and uncle. I signed the guardianship papers without even blinking an eye or shedding a tear. I was severely depressed, totally lacking in emotion— a walking zombie. My aunt, who (along with an uncle) was to assume guardianship of the two eldest kids, later told me that the notary public had to pull her aside because of her concern for me.

My husband, on the other hand, was in survival mode; caving was not an option. He was like a robot, tending very mechanically, yet emotionally, to everything that required his attention (within his ability to do so). Our third and fourth children bounced between a sitter and their aunt and uncle's home, about forty minutes away, who also, very kindly, and sacrificially, took full-time care of their goddaughter, our baby. This care went on for an extended period of time.

Chapter 6

Things Actually Got Worse

(Episode #4)

I had been released or discharged to my own recognizance on July 31, 2001. By my birthday, August 3, I was seriously depressed, but needed to sign the guardianship papers. In that condition, I also needed to try to follow up with psychiatric care after release from that third episode.

I was to follow up with a new psychiatrist on an ongoing out-patient basis, starting with an appointment on August 9th. I am happy to report that somehow, miraculously, I did. My psychiatrist performed an Initial Psychiatric Assessment of me on that day. I would like to say that this was the first out-patient psychiatric visit and the very beginning of my wellness journey. As it happened, though, this was almost the *end* of my journey. I was in a moderate to severe depression and was barely functioning.

Around August 20th, believing I was doing well enough, my aunt called to say that our oldest child needed to be evaluated by the school's Special Education Department. Apparently the oldest had been struggling with attention and focus and was quite often found to be staring off into space. This came as a huge blow. I had home-schooled them and knew that this child was very bright... maybe even gifted. This news sent me spiraling under.

Years ago, Special Education was known for certain stereo-types, and it made me feel as though they were categorizing my child unfairly. My child was likely having transitional, emotional and boredom issues. I felt powerless in the situation, living so far away.

By the next day, everything seemed out of control. My family was strung out everywhere, and I could not help but feel I had caused too much irreversible damage. Everything in me was fighting to stay hopeful, but nothing inside of me was cooperating. I was desperate for peace and serenity, but none would be found. Depression quickly spiraled downward, like a vicious vortex sucking me under.

The next few paragraphs and the medical records that follow concern a suicide attempt. If you're uncomfortable reading this, you can move past the hospital notes.

This next state, in psychiatric terms, is known as suicidal ideation. This is where fleeting thoughts of suicide can worsen and develop into an actual plan. For me, though, I have come to call it suicidal fixation. I was totally content carrying out ANY number of plans, intending FULLY to carry out at least ONE to completion. Then, I began to very anxiously obsess and fixate on taking ALL the meds that were available to me from the past few months of trial and error. I remember looking in the mirror and all I could see was failure; financial, marital, parental, and even spiritual failure.

I would look up to see a full-size poster of the Stations of the Cross on our large bathroom mirror. I reached up, pulled it down, tore it up, and threw it in the trash can. It was not a soul angry or disappointed with Jesus. It was more like a soul saying, "I am so terribly sorry, Jesus".

I took nearly every single pill in sight, in almost every single bottle... soon I would slip away. My husband came home from work and found me in our bedroom convulsing, with plastic bags next to me—I intended to tie them over my head. He called 911 and I was rushed to the hospital, where I remained unconscious for two and a half days.

I have been told that my eldest aunt called my grand-mother, who immediately called another aunt and told her to come over at once. As my aunt arrived at my grandma's house she was told "Aurelia attempted suicide. She's still alive, but you have to go!" My aunt rushed off to the Regional Hospital roughly seventy miles away. She arrived to enter what was a huge room where my eldest aunt was already sitting at my bed-side. My eldest aunt gave her a look that was kind of saying, "No, it doesn't look good."

They were both allowed to stay the night, taking turns with the one comfortable chair in the room. Early in the morning the nurses came, checking on me. I was still out. The two nurses, a man and a woman, were at a table looking over my charts. As my aunt tells me, suddenly the man said, "Oh my God, look at this!"

The lady said, "What?"

And he said, "She saved her own life! She's going to make it!"

He explained to the nurse that several of the pills that I took should have killed me, but that I had also inadvertently taken several other medications that had an antagonistic effect, meaning the medications had essentially canceled each other out, much like an antidote to a poison.

Upon hearing this, my second aunt hurried across the room and said, "What are you talking about? I'm her aunt, I *need* to know what you are talking about!"

The man said, "Yes, you do. We think she has a chance." He told my aunts, "Keep working on her, keep trying to wake her up. Just touch her arm, touch her face, do anything you can."

For the next 6 hours or so they worked on rubbing my head, touching my arms, and generally trying to wake me up. My aunts would say "Wake up Aurelia, wake up. We need to talk to you, Aurelia." All of a sudden, my right eye opened. The second aunt said "Aurelia, you have got to work with us. We need you to wake up. Please, honey, wake up."

I am told that I said, ever so quietly, "I'm trying. I'm trying." And suddenly, I was awake. My aunts say it was like a miracle, largely because they had been praying for one.

Once I was awake, I was taken straight to the Mental Hospital. On my way out the room, I glanced and saw my sibling there, who lived on the east coast. I couldn't make heads or tails of why I was there, or why he was there. I ended up staying at the mental hospital, this time, for a month.

Whenever people inevitably ask the question: "Where were you on September 11, 2001?", I quickly, yet very sadly, go back to this visit to the Mental Hospital.

Suicide is a difficult subject; so many people lose their loved ones to this troublesome taker. Over the years, I have come to know of several people who have committed suicide.

I mostly think of them as snatched up into Heaven, into the arms of our Heavenly Father, relieved of whatever their desperation or mental state, or of whatever their situation or suffering could have possibly been.

HOSPITAL ADMISSION NOTES:

DATE OF ADMISSION: 08/22/01

HISTORY OF PRESENT ILLNESS: This 35-year-old female was found by her husband unresponsive at approximately 1830 on 8/21/01. She was found by a bunch of empty pill bottles.... the patient was recently diagnosed with bipolar disorder in May 2001. She has been hospitalized at a Psychiatric Hospital three times since then, the last time approximately a month ago for about a week. The aunts say she has been alternating between mania and depression. Most recently she has been depressed over the past couple of weeks.... The pill bottles that she was found with are as below:

- Effexor XR 75mg tablets filled 08/20/01 #30 pills; the bottle was empty
- Remeron 45 mg tablets filled 08/20/01 #30 tablets; empty.

- Lorazepam 0.5 mg tablets filled 07/31/01 #60 tablets; empty.
- Zyprexa 10 mg tablets filled 07/31/01 #30 tablets; empty.
- Zyprexa 5 mg tablets filled 07/02/01 #45; 42 left in bottle currently.
- Trazodone 100mg tablets filled on 5/25/01 #30; empty
- Zyprexa 15mg tablets filled on 5/25/01 #30; empty.
- Remeron 30 mg tablets, no date filled on the bottle, apparently 30 pills; empty.

In the emergency room, she had a nasogastric lavage which did lavage out multiple pill fragments, and she was given charcoal.

VITAL SIGNS: Temperature 97.1 on admission. Respiratory rate has been 24 to 28, pulse 105 currently, blood pressure 97/58 and has been as low as 87/55 in the emergency room......

GENERAL: She is an unresponsive female lying in an emergency room cot. She does withdraw to blood draws and moans a little.

LABORATORY: Comprehensive metabolic panel generally normal except for potassium 3.2. CBC shows white count 7.0, hematocrit 42, platelets 249......

PLAN: Admit her to the ICU. Supportive measures......

The Admission History & Mental Status Examination of my fourth Mental Health hospitalization contained information such as:

ADMISSION DATE: 8/24/01

PATIENT INFORMATION: Aurelia Roybal is a 35-year-old married female, admitted status post serious suicide attempt for her fourth psychiatric hospitalization here in the past year.

HISTORY OF PRESENT ILLNESS: The patient had a post-partum onset of psychosis following the birth of her fifth child this past year. The patient has had difficulty with increasing psychosis and manic mania since that time. The patient has been on multiple medications recently. She states that she has been sleeping up to 12 hours a day; she is very frustrated by being unable to get anything done in regard to house chores. She also has been non-compliant with her medications and took an overdose of all her medication.... on August 21st. The patient likely took the overdose sometime around 3 o'clock in the afternoon. She was found by her husband at 6:30. She required charcoal and lavage. She was hospitalized for three days for medical stabilization and brought here for further evaluation and treatment.

MENTAL STATUS EXAMINATION: At the time of admission the patient is alert and oriented. She has good eye contact. She has a depressed mood with a restricted affect. She currently denies psychosis, though she tends to be somewhat hyper-religious and grandiose in her thought processes and content. Her judgment is fair. She has ongoing suicidal ideation. She denies any homicidal ideation. Patient has intact judgment and insight.

IMPRESSION: (DSM-IV):

Axis I.   Bipolar affective disorder, with current depression, status post suicide attempt.

Axis II.   No diagnosis.

Axis III.   Status post serious overdose attempt.

Axis IV.   Psychosocial stressors: Moderate.

Axis V.   GAF currently rated at 25.

INITIAL TREATMENT PLAN/RECOMMENDATIONS: We will consider a trial of ECT in order to help with mood stabilization in this patient who has had over four hospitalizations in the past year.

I want to emphasize that just because you are released from a mental hospital, doesn't mean you are out of the woods; in fact, you could still become a danger to yourself or to others, especially without proper follow-up and care.

In that month, after much investigation and deliberation made by family on my behalf, it was decided that I would undergo treatments of Electro Convulsive Therapy (ECT). ECT is electrical current applied to the brain of an anesthetized person. It is used to treat severe depression. The patient would have electrodes placed on their head and small currents or electrical pulses would be delivered to pass through the brain in order to initiate a brief seizure. It can reverse certain mental health conditions/symptoms such as depression.

In total, I was given six separate treatments. Fortunately for me, the procedure had advanced substantially, and a more modern version was available than what was available only decades prior. Far enough back in the day, a much cruder treatment, and quite possibly even an asylum could have easily been a part of my reality. Thanks to modern medicine, I would soon be released.

Speaking very quickly to the ECT, if it were to become necessary once more, I would do it again without much reservation, although new treatments and advancements are always forthcoming. My longest-lasting side-effect has indeed been memory issues. I experience extremely poor retention and recall. At times, my memory seems mostly unreliable, making work and general reminiscing intensely challenging. Other times, my memory can be semi-decent to good. At best, I would say that my memory is random and unpredictable. I would trade that any day for the much-improved quality of life that I now enjoy. I have no regrets with the decision made on my behalf and in my *essential absence*!

By late September, we needed to figure out how on earth to face the music. How does one focus on gradually getting better while immediately needing to get their family back together and tend to them as well? This turned out to be *a lot harder* than you could ever imagine. In hindsight, and with the healing nature of time, we can now somehow manage to laugh, even though deep inside we still basically cringe and nearly cry, just thinking about some of the things that happened during that intensely wild and challenging time in our lives.

During that summer, the kids got head lice (my poor immediate and extended family). It already seemed hard enough to deal with all that was going on already, much less add to that, having to treat the whole family for head lice! In that same summer, a box of cereal was left open. My husband, his sister, and two of our sons were having breakfast, when it was discovered that the mouthful about to be taken by our son had worms! What was worse, was that my husband had already eaten an entire bowlful!! It sounds disgusting, but more than that, it speaks to an overwhelmed bunch of people just trying to get by.

Chapter 7

My Physical & Mental Health at War

(Episode #5)

It took some time to get used to a new schedule that would include weekly visits with my psychiatrist, maintaining prescription refills, and taking my meds nightly, but I was finally on the road to being considered compliant! My psychiatrist recommended a psychologist for me to see, and I saw her weekly. According to her notes, I started sessions with her on October 3, 2001.

As I understand it, by Winter Break of 2001, we were rejoined together as a family, except for our baby. The baby was extremely well-cared for, as I am told, for about an entire year or so by her godparents. We are so blessed to have had their help. Most who have helped us will never know how much we appreciate their support. Unfortunately, we have never been in the best condition to manage anything more than just keeping on, much less thanking everyone properly. This still holds true today, even though I am mostly regulated and considered stable. We hope that each person involved realizes this has brought us quite literally to our knees... which is right where God probably wanted us.

During that Winter Break, we felt it necessary to spend some quality time with the kids, so we took a road trip to Las Vegas, Nevada. We had the time-share, after all! The kids were eager to be together, and in general, because of all the love and care they were given, seemed rather resilient and virtually unscathed.

After returning home in January of 2002, we were to put the three oldest in Public School. Home-schooling no longer seemed practical. In fact, it would have been considered irresponsible and, quite possibly, an outrage!

The oldest was to be enrolled to continue in second grade, and our second oldest continued with kindergarten. Our middle child would join me when I volunteered in the kindergarten classroom on the weekdays that my husband did not work. It took time, but life slowly started to normalize.

By the fall of 2002, when the new school year had begun, I was beginning to function better. We had the three oldest kids in second grade, first grade and kindergarten. Once again, we were barely handling life, but we were managing better than we had been in the summer of 2001.

We felt it important to socialize the kids, so we put the kids in soccer in the 2003 season with much needed help from their great-aunt (the one that I had previously called 911 on). Originally, there were three practices for three teams for the three oldest kids, who were of age. Later, we were able to put two of the kids on one team, leaving us with *only* two practices with only two teams, meaning only two games on Saturdays.

Then, in September of 2004, misfortune struck. I was exhausted all the time and was taking naps at every opportunity. My health was jeopardized by a condition which would later be found to be menorrhagia, or abnormally heavy bleeding at menstruation. I had always had heavy cycles, but this was largely a cumulative effect met with excessively larger flows.

I began to behave questionably and was decompensating or deteriorating rapidly. I think this was the episode where everything I was experiencing seemed to be in fast motion, however, everyone and everything around me seemed to be going in slow motion. Honestly speaking, the fast-motion/slow-motion bit was downright hilarious, almost like in a cartoon or something. I felt like a marionette master! It was as if I was in control and running circles around everybody. Truth be told, I was extremely far from being in control of anything at all.

I went *voluntarily* to the emergency room, because we were quite certain it was a manic episode in the making. A slightly more educated, more experienced person was now trying her best to be responsible and cooperative. As it had turned out, it was a serious case of anemia causing everything. I was given two blood transfusions and was released shortly thereafter. I felt like an escape artist or a jail bird (what with leaving the ER and avoiding a mental-health hospitalization). I could not believe I was free to go without Haldol or restraints! I had already become rather familiar with that whole routine, so, I guess I was pleased to be sent home.

About a week later, I ended up back in the Mental Hospital. This was likely the episode where I counted (shouting) backward from a number that sounded like my husband's name, and then rapidly counted down the numbers—nine, eight, seven, six, five, four, three, two, one, shouted my husband's name in sheer desperation, just to start the countdown again. I repeated this several times. Each time I got closer to the number one, I felt like I was going to die! I was in a heightened panicked state, severely manic.

This time, after the routine ER visit, however, I ended up admitted to unfamiliar surroundings. The hospital I had become accustomed to was no longer serving the adult population. They were only treating adolescents. I ended up at the University Hospital nearby. I was admitted for 2 weeks. I had visited my mom and two siblings at this hospital on different admissions in the years prior to my own diagnosis. Visiting and staying, however, are two completely different experiences. Everything was new to me.

The following Admission Note summarizes my admission to the University Mental Hospital:

ATTENDING ADMISSION NOTE
Wednesday, September 22, 2004

D: I have seen the patient, reviewed the chart, and agree with the resident's assessment and plan.

History of Present Illness: The patient is a 38-year-old Hispanic female with bipolar disorder, who had been stable for three years until the past week. She was taken to the nearby Regional Medical Center by her family on Monday night for escalating symptoms of mania, including psychomotor agitation, increased activity and cleaning, decreased p.o. intake and increased verbosity. She had also reportedly barricaded her eldest child in the bathroom, at which point 911 was called. The patient was evaluated at the outside hospital and deemed to need admission. As they had no bed, she was transferred. Prior to the transfer, she was medicated with Haldol: 10 mg and Ativan: 2 mg. She was very sedated and remained sedated until this morning, sleeping throughout the night. The patient states that she did not really need to be in the hospital but acknowledges that she has been deteriorating. She reports being very tired and having a multitude of social stressors going on. She states that she has been taking her medications as prescribed. She reports, however, that last week she was noted to be anemic and was transfused, two units, in the Emergency Room. Because of her ongoing fatigue, her psychiatrist had started her on Lamotrigine in May and had recently completed a taper off Lithium.

Past Psychiatric History is notable for a diagnosis of Bipolar affective disorder. The patient has a history of mania, followed by depression, requiring a course of ECT. The patient, in the past, has been hospitalized in another Mental Health hospital and is currently followed with her outpatient psychiatrist. Her last hospitalizations were in 2001. She also had a suicide attempt by overdose at that time. She has been stable as an outpatient since then.

Family Psychiatric History is notable for bipolar disorder in multiple family members, including the patient's mother, two of her [siblings] and a cousin. There are no completed suicides.

Substance History: There is no alcohol or drug use

Medical History: is notable for hypothyroidism, with the patient's TSH at her primary care physician on 09.09.04 being 6.8. The patient was recently diagnosed with a severe iron deficiency anemia, probably secondary to menorrhagia. The patient had a documented hematocrit of 34 in 07.02 and on 09.09.04, her hematocrit was 27.

Review of Systems is notable for chronic headaches, that started in the past year and heavy periods.

Allergies: Depakote, which caused a rash.

Mental Status Examination: On my examination, the patient is a well-developed, thin and pale-appearing Hispanic female, who is neatly groomed and dressed. Her behavior is calm. Her affect is constricted and at times she is slightly elevated and at other near tears. Mood is, "I guess I'm manic." Speech is pressured and difficult to direct. Thought process shows circumstantiality, over-inclusiveness and flight of ideas, with tangentiality at times. Thought content is unremarkable with there being no evidence of grandiosity or delusions. The patient denies any hallucinations and denies any thoughts of harming herself or others. Vegetative symptoms include decreased sleep and appetite and increased energy. Insight is adequate in some ways in that the patient acknowledges that she has bipolar disorder, is currently manic and needs medication. Judgment appears, at times, to be impaired by her mania.

A: 38-year-old female with bipolar disorder, becoming slowly manic over the past several weeks with markedly increased symptoms for three days prior to admission and with significant medical problems concurrently as well as significant social problems.

AXIS I   Bipolar AFFECTIVE DISORDER, MANIC, SEVERE.

AXIS II   NONE.

AXIS III HYPOTHYROIDISM; IRON DEFICIENCY ANE-
MIA, PROBABLE SECONDARY TO MENORRHAGIA.

AXIS IV   STRESSORS: SEVERE, PROBLEMS WITH
CHRONIC ILLNESS; PRIMARY SUPPORT GROUP; FI-
NANCIAL.

AXIS V   20

While in the Mental Hospital, I was incredibly stressed out about finances. So much so that I spent the better part of my admittance on the phone with Social Security. I was told that I would not qualify. Also, the 'Children, Youth and Families Department' got involved, which had me beside myself.

A cousin of mine came to visit. He came during a mean game of kick the dry-erase marker cap across the floor (much like hockey, only with our feet) that another patient and I were involved in. I was easily distracted, and very bored. He probably had to wonder where my priorities were, but I knew better. He comes from a family of extreme love. Over the years, my whole life really, their family has been a pillar of love and support.

This goes for both sides of my family. Sometimes, I could not help but feel that the lack that was experienced by my brothers and me growing up, was observed at times directly and indirectly by extended family over the course of our youth. This, I feel, was compensated by all who loved us. We have, in my mind, been given much compassion and have been very well loved!

Although edible, the food at this hospital was very heavy in carbs and fats. As mentioned before, putting on weight was a serious struggle for me, and the food was not helping. Due to med changes, I put on weight very rapidly, but had a heck of a time taking it off. Over the years, I put on ten to fifteen pounds almost each episode/med-change. I have kept on roughly three to five pounds per episode/med-change that I could not successfully take off. I originally weighed about 145 to 150 in 2001, and at my highest I have weighed about 195. In recent years I have been fluctuating between 175 and 185, with this past year or so being my most challenging, sitting at about 190.

Taking meds is no party, but it has proven to me to be worthwhile in the grand scheme of things. Although side-effects are rough and sometimes hard to handle, the meds keep me balanced and are worth every obstacle.

The following Discharge Summary summarizes the two-week admission at the University Mental Hospital:

DISCHARGE SUMMARY:

DATE OF ADMISSION: 9/21/04

DATE OF DISCHARGE: 10/05/04

DISCHARGE DIAGNOSIS:

AXIS I   Bipolar AFFECTIVE DISORDER, TYPE I, MOST RECENT EPISODE MANIC, *Severe*

AXIS II   DEFERRED

AXIS III   HYPOTHYROIDISM; *Fe Deficiency Anemia*

AXIS IV   SOCIAL; PRIMARY SUPPORT; FINANCIAL

AXIS V   55

ADMISSION HISTORY:

This is a 38-year-old female with a history of Bipolar Affective Disorder, type I, who was brought in by her husband. The
patient had reportedly been stable on Lithium for a long time,
then discontinued it secondary to diarrhea. The patient had
been manic for about three days with manic behavior that
has been progressively escalating. The patient has had, for
the last couple of weeks, increased cleaning, agitation, talking,
decreased eating, and ended with the barricading of her child
in the bathroom, although patient had been treated and sent
home with outpatient follow-up. The patient's symptoms continued to escalate again three days ago, and she was brought
back for evaluation.

LABORATORY DATA:

CBC was significant for WBCs 30.9, RBCs of 5.4, MCV of 70,
RDW of 25.4%

Chemistry 7 was within normal limits.

Liver function tests were significant for an albumin of 5.2.

Urine was positive for ketones of 15, squamous epithelial
cells of 6, otherwise, was within normal limits

Urine pregnancy test was negative.

Thyroid was 11.5.

Lithium level on September 25, 2004 was 0.3. On October 1,
2004 it was 0.8

Urine tox was positive for benzodiazepines.

HOSPITAL COURSE:

Bipolar Affective Disorder, Most Recent Episode Mania:
The patient initially wanted to be discharged right away, denying that she had very many manic symptoms. However, with

continued talk therapy, patient was able to see that her symptoms were fairly acute and recognized that she was needing to stay in the hospital. Her insight to her illness was especially remarkable as she was able to, for the most part, recognize the rapid speech, the flight of ideas, and the goal-directed behavior. The patient was very compliant with her medications and was willing to take and increase them as needed.

She was restarted on the Lithium Citrate at 300 mg b.i.d. Her Effexor was slowly tapered from her outpatient dose of 225mg, down to 37.5 mg until she is off the medication completely. Since patient had been stable on her anti-depressant and her mood stabilizer as an outpatient, initially it was thought that she would just decrease the dose to prevent her depression from recurring. However, it was found despite efforts to decrease her Effexor gradually and to maintain mood stabilizer, she was just not able to "come down fast enough," so Effexor was tapered off. Lamictal had been started as an outpatient as well and was gradually increased to 200 mg, p.o. q. day; patient tolerated this dose well.

By discharge, the patient had a reduction in manic behaviors. She did tend to pace and have a lot of propensity for being active. She did, however, no longer have as high an activity level as on admission. She was speaking in much more normal rate. She did have an elevated mood, but it was not a manic or euphoric mood. She denied any delusions of any voices or psychotic thoughts. The patient's husband was willing to take her home and she had significant support awaiting her at discharge. Things to be managed by outpatient doctor: The patient was discharged on Effexor XR 37.5 mg, p.o. q. day and this should be tapered off by outpatient psychiatrist, and at some point, reinstated as clinically indicated. The patient should have her Lithium level checked again in six weeks to monitor her level. She was also told to maintain the same amount of salt intake as she normally does and to drink the same amount of fluids as she normally does to avoid fluctuations in Lithium levels.

Hypothyroidism:

The patient's TSH was significantly elevated and she was re-started on Synthroid 0.150 mg, q. day without any problems.

Anemia from Iron Deficiency:

Based on patient's laboratories, it appears that she has had iron deficiency anemia for quite some time, most likely secondary to extremely heavy periods and multiple pregnancies close together in time. Patient was seen by an OB-GYN physician during her hospitalization. At that visit, OB-GYN performed a pap smear by manual examination and an endometrial biopsy. The patient will have follow-up visits with OB-GYN as an outpatient. Recommendations are to start some sort of hormone therapy as patient is Catholic and has strong views of oral contraception. OB-GYN and patient were going to work together to find an option that would be satisfactory to their religious beliefs.

Legal:

Because patient had put her child at risk and Police Department was called because of her behaviors, CYFD was notified that there may be a possible risk of harm to patient's children as she has five, very small children. The patient and patient's husband are aware that CYFD was notified.

DISCHARGE DISPOSITION:

The patient was discharged home to family. She had significant family support to assist with housework and bills and plans to modify their financial situation were in place already at the time of discharge.

Discharge Medications:

Ferrous Sulphate: 3 times a day with food
Synthroid: 0.150 mg. q. day
Citrucel: 1 heaping teaspoon in 8 ounces of water
Lithium Citrate: 600 mg, twice a day with food
Lamictal: 300 mg, a day with food
Temazepam: 15mg, at bedtime
Effexor XR: 37.5 mg q. day

Follow-up:
The patient has an appointment with a family counselor on November 2, 2004 at 5:45 pm

The patient has an outpatient appointment with her psychiatrist on Tuesday, October 12 at 9:40 am

The patient has a counseling/therapy appointment with her psychologist on Tuesday, October 12 at 3:15 pm

The patient has a Primary Care appointment with her Physician on October 6, 2004 at 10:30 am

CONDITION OF PATIENT UPON DISCHARGE:
The patient is considered to be of low risk of harm to herself or others at the time of discharge. She denied any suicidal or homicidal ideation and she has been compliant with her medications and is willing to cooperate with physicians and family to maintain safety. She is capable of making her own medication and financial decisions on her own.

Since my health was primary to my Bipolar, I was given an appointment to see an Obstetrician and Gynecologist during my admission to address the menorrhagia and birth control. After my fourth episode in 2001, we had chosen Natural Family Planning (NFP) and had succeeded with that method of birth control. The doctor spoke to me about other options. One option that came highly recommended and was considered as medically necessary, was a partial hysterectomy (meaning the removal of the uterus with the keeping of my ovaries). This would not put me into menopause. This is what I opted for. It was not scheduled until February of 2005.

There were generally pluses and minuses to being in the Mental Hospital each time. One plus each time, was the opportunity to get balanced and to get rest. One minus, this time, was missing my Goddaughter's Baptism in New Hampshire. Fortunately, another plus was being able to make it to my brother's wedding, which I was able to attend by the skin of my teeth. They were married only days after I was discharged.

In fact, a cousin came to help me pick out clothes and iron them for the wedding. I will never forget some advice she had for me: "You've got to stop folding everyone's underwear." Sounds silly, perhaps, to those who don't know me and who didn't know our situation, but in general, I took it as a loving message of concern for me to lessen my load and to simplify wherever I could. Sometime thereafter, I migrated to not folding and putting their laundry away at all. I washed and dried and promptly laid flat the family's laundry. This saved me unknown bunches of time over the years. That one act of love was deeply appreciated and was one of many still to follow.

I was discharged on October 5, 2004. Several things happened in the months that followed that led us to move back to the town we grew up in. One thing was that on Ash Wednesday, February 9, 2005, the kids had either catechism or church children's choir practice, but they also were to have a talent show at their elementary school (K- 6) that evening.

Our ten-year-old was to play the Titanic theme song, "My Heart Will Go On" on the keyboard, and our eight-year-old was to sing "El Shaddai", a praise song. We went home between events to get the kids dressed and ready. I needed to iron their clothing and curl my daughter's hair. Meanwhile, I put a big pot of water on the stove and began to boil pasta, as I was going to prepare tuna salad for dinner after the show. We went to the talent show without realizing the pasta was still on the stove.

When we arrived nearly two hours later, we were welcomed to a house full of thick, awful smoke. The pasta was hardly recognizable; it had turned into something like a round-shaped charcoal brick.

The insurance company called it a protein fire and had to put us up in a hotel, in two adjacent rooms, for two or more weeks. Unfortunately, I was scheduled for the hysterectomy within that timeframe and had to recover during that stay.

While we were there, my brother and sister-in-law approached us with a proposition to move back to our hometown, with the possibility that we would have more support. After much consideration, we moved back home in May 2005, once the school year ended.

The goal was simple: keep taking care of myself as best as possible and know that there were plenty of people who could help if it ever became necessary.

Chapter 8

The Sleepwalking Incident

(Episode #6)

Like any of our previous moves, we had lots of help moving all our "stuff." Although the home we moved from seemed smaller, and the home we moved into seemed bigger, we found ourselves unable to move everything in. We had a large, covered porch full of unopened boxes, and a large pile of boxes (mostly full of books) covered with a heavy-duty tarp outside. My brother showed my husband how to build a shed, and over the course of my husband's next sabbatical, with the help of my brother, we were able to sufficiently store most of our "stuff".

From May 2005 to July 2007, my husband still worked in the city we formerly lived in, roughly eighty miles away. Since we still had the apartments, he generally stayed there at a friend's house all week, plus part of the weekend, in order to do apartment maintenance. I was roughly running the show at home alone. This took a toll on me. It came with many challenges, hence: anxiety, overwhelm, and exhaustion. Sound familiar?

We were not unlike many families. We, too, had our share of drama and challenges within the family. During the 2005-2006 school year, attempting to be proactive in avoiding any chance of hospitalization, we had two of our children go to live with my brother and sister-in-law that lived just a few miles away. They attended most, if not all the school year while living there with them.

In 2006, I began to file applications for disability despite having been told that we would not qualify previously. This was difficult due to battles with my physical health (asthma), fragile mental health, and an overall sense of overwhelm. An example of paperwork overload included some of the paperwork given to us in May 2001 (upon discharge from the first episode, apparently). This was paperwork given to us to file for disability, but somehow it got lost in the shuffle. I did not find some of that paperwork until very recently, when searching through records and doing research for writing this book (2019/2020).

In September 2006, I completed a FUNCTION REPORT – ADULT for the Social Security Administration. The following bullets are excerpts taken from that form:

- I'm generally up by 7:00 (exhausted) get kids off to school bus by 8:00, randomly, consistently, predictably spend entire day tending to laundry, housekeeping, mail, bills, phone calls, and almost always get very little accomplished. Kids off bus at 4:30. Dinner between 4:30 and 5:00, chores, homework, baths, bedtime, other demands, bed between 10:00 – 11:00 (w/sleep meds if 11:00 pm or later or if too wound up mentally, emotionally, etc.). Generally, fight off nap daily otherwise it ends up being anywhere from 2-4 hours and extremely difficult to wake from.

- I find it difficult managing my home and family because of meds, difficulty w/sleep, handling stress, and battling with exhaustion
- I take sleep meds as needed (about 3-4 nights a week because my gears are turning, and I can't fall asleep on my own and can't function anymore without at least 8-9 hours of sleep.
- My husband handles half or more of what I used to. I'm generally overwhelmed, exhausted, fuzzy-headed, forgetful, and he's needed to.
- I don't really have passion for anything anymore. I prioritize my family, my health, and am pretty much consumed by both.
- I struggle with details & recollection.
- Since my illness, I have come to realize that certain boundaries, due to stressors, have been necessary.
- I have a very difficult time following/focusing on even casual conversation...
- I have a huge challenge with concentration, focus, and reading (I have always had problems with reading) but now it is much worse. I do well w/one instruction at a time if not complex or detailed. Things just seem to go in one ear and out the other. I seem to have a problem w/ retention and recollection and often have to ask things over and over.
- My regimen has had ongoing change (especially related to energy and mood) over past 5 years.
- Challenges have been ongoing and still not resolved pertaining to poor energy, mood, stress.
- Housework has piled up, bills to collection, credit scores dropped, finances a wreck, the house a disaster zone, sick and tired all the time, etc.

- I went from being an enthusiastic, passionate, loving, caring, personable, and sociable wife and mother to an awful, sad, miserable, depleted, confused, ashamed, baffled and bewildered one, and to a desperate zombie (referencing the timeframe between Episodes 2 and 3). It was against my morals and values and beliefs (suicide), but I was not in my own healthy right mind.
- The past 5 years have been a living hell in so many ways. We've endured a dramatic reversal in our finances/economic well-being. We have suffered devastating consequences due to decisions that were made during the periods of mania.

* * *

By January 2007, I had essentially gathered and created a chaotic mess. If it were not for my aunt getting involved at the level that she did (including obtaining records, organizing and reviewing documentation, communication back and forth with the Social Security Administration, and the hiring of a Disability Attorney), I would not have been awarded Social Security Disability Income, period. The process is so complicated and so daunting that it is a huge challenge for a person with mental illness to navigate on their own.

I was doing my best to apply for SSDI but was doing a rather poor job of it at best. I was stressed out, overwhelmed, and not handling things very well. My aunt observed how chaotic things were and offered to become my legal advocate. We needed the records from previous hospital visits to show evidence of my diagnosis, but a huge problem arose. The hospital had closed since I was admitted there in 2001, and we did not know what had happened to my records.

Thus, she began the hunt. She managed to find a woman who had owned the records, but for whatever reasons had decided to sell them. Long story short, they had eventually been sold to a man who had moved to Florida. My aunt got in contact with him and learned that the records were still at a facility in our state. Although he gave his permission to have the records accessed, it was past 5pm and it was too late to phone the facility before the weekend.

Anyhow, my aunt was part-owner of a bed and breakfast, and would serve breakfast each morning. Whenever she was done serving the guests, she would facilitate introductions asking their first name, the kind of work they did, and where they were from. When one man's turn came up, he said he was from our neighboring city and that he worked for that facility where my records were!!

In shock, my aunt said, "What?"

He said, "I work at [name of facility]. It's a business where we keep records."

She offered to comp his night for his assistance in finding my records. Some time elapsed and he said, "Ok, Ma'am, I'd be happy to help you, but it won't do any good for me to help you tomorrow. We have to do it today!"

She then said, "Today is Sunday!"

And he says "I know! But we are burning the records to-morrow!" It would seem the destruction date was at hand, which meant that legally the records had to be destroyed.

They put their heads together, called his boss, two ladies were asked to go in and pull the records and make copies on a Sunday, paperwork was filed, and the records had to be picked up (seventy miles away) before 7am the following morning. My aunt declared she would be there at 6am, and she and a friend were successful!

It wouldn't have happened other than for the morning introductions! Thanks of course to my aunt and our friend persevering in the hunt, and thanks be to God for always coming through. The records would not have been obtained without some *major coincidences*, or as I prefer to call them, "my own personal and incredible little miracles." God has taken very good care of me.

These records not only came in handy during the Disability Determination Process, but even now, in being able to reference my records in order to write this book. Getting these was only the first step in getting my Disability, though. Now we needed to find out if I qualified based on the records and other information. This is where another "little" miracle happened.

My aunt had done some research, which revealed that 20 quarters were required with a required minimum income per quarter in order to fulfill qualification. After some investigation, my aunt (and our friend who worked for her) discovered that I had 19 ¾ quarters. I was just shy of qualifying. They went through my papers again, and found my resignation letter, which was dated April 1, 1996. However, in the body of the letter they found that it stated the effective date as April 11, 1996. I was paid through April 11, 1996 and had enough workdays to have earned enough to satisfy that 20th quarter!

Roughly, around 2006, before streaming apps were out, I made it through by watching episodes of *I Love Lucy* and *Seventh Heaven*. Surprisingly, distracting the mind is helpful when anxious (light-hearted television, mainly comedies and family-oriented programming did the trick for me!). Although helpful, this was certainly more of a Band-Aid than a remedy. It pacified me for a bit, but it certainly was not a cure. What ailed me most was *my mind.* I was overly anxious and highly dissatisfied with my homemaking and parenting in general.

The summer of 2007 was quite challenging in terms of handling my anxiety, my stress, and my health. By this next episode, (my sixth), July 17th, the kids were thirteen, eleven, ten, eight, and six years of age, and all were living at home. What happened this time around was incredibly sad. The kids were on summer break, and I had always had the challenge of having the kids home for break, as we couldn't afford camps or summer programs.

My saving grace was that the kids loved electronics. They occupied themselves a bit outdoors by playing on the trampoline, riding scooters, etc., but mostly, they loved being on the computer or gaming station or being on handheld devices. The kids also liked reading books and all loved our pets. These were enormously helpful in raising our family.

When one has bipolar disorder, the experience of having anxiety or depression, can make it hard to function normally. When one experiences *both together*, it is even harder— remember that having both anxiety and depression can often be the makings of a mixed episode.

I was mostly an anxiety-filled nervous wreck until my husband returned home each week. For me, anxiety can feel like your insides are on your outsides. It can feel like you are being wrung out, and like you are a jittery mess. It often would bring me literally to my knees in prayer. Anything could have set my anxiety off, but one event I remember clearly was when our van needed the transmission replaced. A dear friend who was a mechanic came to change the transmission. It was necessary to rig up a jack of sorts for our van, and the whole event was more than I could handle as my mind blew the dangers of the event out of proportion. I couldn't even handle minimal stressors at that time, much less anything extraordinary.

I was also depressed with situations in general (finances, housework, family dynamics, etc.). My husband was gone more than he was home, and the kids were still in need of parenting and interaction. I felt that I was doing an incredibly poor job of it all and was slipping into a deepening depression.

The next few paragraphs concern a suicide attempt and you may want to skip over them if you are in the least bit squeamish. Instead, you can move forward past the next hospital notes.

Several stressors had mounted up during early July, until I was having suicidal ideation. One day we took the kids to the Wellness Center nearby to play and kill some time. I packed a knife in my pocket, and had every intention of using it, but somehow, luckily, I could not easily slip away and do it.

That night though, on July 17th, without my husband having any idea, I stashed a single-edge razor blade by my bed, took my medicine, and hoped I would not wake up until morning. Unfortunately, I woke in the middle of the night with *vicious* suicidal ideation. I was in a stupor. I was heavily medicated, and likely sleepwalking to boot. I was semi-alert and semi-asleep. Only later would I discover that a side-effect of that sleep med was sleepwalking.

I went to the bathroom where I poured a bath. I stepped into the tub and sat down. I took the single-edge razor and proceeded to cut away. I have no idea whether I started on my neck or on my wrists. I remember feeling on my neck for a pulse and aiming for that area. At some point, I remember waking up to sitting in the tubful of pinkish water. When I awoke, it was with a start. It felt urgent now that I needed to finish what I started.

I put on a robe and went to the kitchen for one of the knives that always cut me. Somehow my husband woke up; he was in shock and in total disbelief. He immediately called 911. I fought for my meds for the purpose of overdosing, but it was too late. First responders arrived.

This is the one ambulance ride I have no memory of. I was probably given Haldol or similar. Next thing I knew, I was waking up while they were stitching my wrist at the hospital. Likely, they administered more medicine, as I remember nothing more.

The following is the Discharge Summary from the Regional Medical Center's Behavioral Health Unit Eight-day admission:

DATE OF ADMISSION: 07/17/2007

DATE OF DISCHARGE: 07/24/07

HISTORY OF PRESENT ILLNESS:

This is a 40-year-old married female, mother of 5, with history of bipolar disorder, followed by her psychiatrist in (name of another city). The patient is admitted to the emergency department after presenting with lacerations on her wrist and neck. The patient presents with a chief complaint of "I wasn't handling the pressure at home."

This is a 40-year-old female with a history of Bipolar illness. The patient lives in [name of community]. The patient has 5 children, ages 7, 8.5, 10, 11.5, and 13. The patient's husband works as a technician at [name of company] in [name of city]. He works 12-hour shifts. The patient states that she is left dealing with the kids for summer. [One of the patient's children] has Asperger's Syndrome and also has ADD. [Another] child is diagnosed with ADD. The patient is finding it difficult to cope with her children. The patient also states that they have financial problems. The patient on the day of the overdose woke up at 1:30 in the morning and had thoughts of wanting to hurt herself. The patient made lacerations to her wrists and her neck and laid down in the bathtub. The patient was found by her husband at 4:30 in the morning. The patient's husband called 911. The patient was subsequently admitted to [hospital name]'s Behavioral Health Unit for stabilization.

LABORATORY DATA AT THE TIME OF ADMISSION

Hemoglobin A1C is at 5.14. CMP is significant for an elevated glucose of 164 and elevated bilirubin of 2.1. Chemistries on July 17 showed an elevated sodium of 160, elevated chloride of 127, and albumin of 5.1. Urinalysis was within normal limits. TSH is at 0.03. Cardiac injury panel is within normal limits. Urine pregnancy is negative. CBC with diff is significant for elevated _____ of 35.9 and elevated absolute neutrophil count of 7.9. Urine tox was negative.

HOSPITAL COURSE

The patient is admitted to psychiatry. The patient is continued on her medications, which include Effexor XR 75 mg and Abilify 5mg. The patient was placed on suicide precautions. The patient presented with depressive symptoms, feelings of hopelessness and helplessness, and feeling overwhelmed. The patient's Effexor dose was gradually increased to 225 mg and the patient's Abilify dose was raised to 10mg. The patient's main stressors are her children. The patient has 5 young children; 2 of them have psychiatric diagnoses. The patient needs help in caretaking of these kids. Family sessions were done with the husband, her brother and her aunt. The plan is for her family to take in these kids temporarily until summer vacation is over. This will give the patient a break for about a month. The patient reports significant improvement in mood. The patient complained of insomnia, which was addressed with Trazodone 75mg at bedtime. The patient's plan is to go to a monastery or go to her aunt's home for a short period of time. The patient is denying suicidality. The patient is willing to follow up with her psychiatrist and her therapist in (name of another city)

DISCHARGE MEDICATIONS

1. Effexor XR 225 mg daily
2. Abilify 10 mg daily.
3. Trazodone 75 mg at bedtime

FOLLOWUP

The patient will follow up with her psychiatrist. The patient has an appointment on July 27, 2007 at 12:30. The patient will also follow up with her therapist/psychologist for one-on-one therapy. The patient is encouraged to seek more frequent one-on-one sessions with her.

FINAL DIAGNOSES

Axis I: Bipolar Affective Disorder type 1, most recent episode depressed.

Axis II: Deferred.

Axis III: Status post superficial lacerations to her wrist and neck, hypothyroidism, and status post hysterectomy.

Axis IV: Chronic illness, financial issues.

Axis V: 50

As you would guess, and as my admission/discharge record above state, I ended up in a Mental Hospital— the third facility to date. This time, family intervened on my behalf, and decisions were made that were in my best interest but were not easy to accept. Once I was out of the Mental Hospital, I stayed at an aunt's house. I did not return home for several months. This was intended, I believe, to give me some time to sort things out, and a chance to move toward recovery. This time apart was meant to serve as respite (time for rest, reflection and decompression). Unfortunately, at the time, it also felt a bit like a severe consequence.

My aunt was very generous to open her home to me... although since that time, she has admitted she felt a little concerned as to whether I was still suicidal because of knives, etc. around her house. Minutes turned to hours, hours to days, days turned to weeks, and weeks turned into months. I still choose to take time for respite.

Recovery from each episode, at least from my own experience, can take months, and cumulatively, may even take many years. In essence, some of the experiences, setbacks, memories, and even some of the stories regarding one's behavior can be difficult to work past. I liken it to digging a hole. The deeper you dig, the harder it is to throw out the dirt. A dear friend of mine once told me "All you can do is try your best, and that has got to be good enough."

I went on walks and called my cousin almost daily. I remember the phone calls, but hardly remember the conversations. It meant so much to have my cousin's support. So much was jeopardized and so much seemed so unstable and vulnerable. It helped talking to someone regularly. Walking has been such a blessing to me over the years. Even in the Mental Hospitals I "paced", not only for exercise, but to keep from being bored to death.

I highly recommend exercise as part of a normal routine of living with this disorder. The benefits are plentiful: 1) better health and fitness; 2) exercise naturally aids in the quality and quantity of sleep; and 3) decompression (time to think and/or organize thoughts).

By nature, though, I was somewhat high-strung. It wasn't long before I was increasing my schedule just due to the sheer nature of having five kids. The older ones were in a special, free tennis program that summer, and it was necessary to take them to and from practice. It was hard "letting go" of so much for so long, especially at these ages.

In pretty short order, my aunt learned of a program given by the National Alliance for the Mentally Ill (NAMI) that was advertised in the newspaper called Family to Family. She, my husband, my brother and my sister- in-law would begin attending classes soon after.

I do not remember how, but I discovered a Bipolar Group being held downtown in the city where I stayed with my aunt. I began attending this group in August of 2007. It is sad but true that, since I hardly read, this was where I finally started to learn more about Bipolar.

The LPCC, (Licensed Professional Clinical Counselor), who ran the Bipolar Group is the same counselor with whom I currently attend Bipolar Group (more than thirteen years later!), and with whom I have had Individual Therapy with (for a slightly lesser period).

I attended the weekly Bipolar Group each Friday. I felt very welcome, without judgment, and *uncomfortable* all at the same time. At the beginning, I had to grapple with whether I felt like I belonged with "*those people*".

I was struggling with the idea of identifying/relating with others who had mental illness. I was judging.

As it has turned out, "*those people*" have enriched my life greatly, and I am indebted to each person I have encountered who has courageously and generously shared different aspects of their journeys, so that others might also benefit. It took some humbling and submission of ego to get to a point that I could truly receive and contribute at a level that was no longer judgmental or selfish.

The group was a safe environment of peers gathered to share, vent, and process difficult things of all sorts. One veteran member shared that the group served as her "safety net." She could rely on the group to monitor her energy, activity, and behavior to avoid any likelihood of an episode. This was true not just for her, but for many that attended.

There is power in relating to people who also have similar experiences, helpful insights, and useful feedback. Sometimes we act and feel like we know it all, but there is always plenty to learn and plenty of ego worth shedding.

Don't get me wrong, professionals are seriously needed and are invaluable. They have their hearts, minds, and objectives in the right place, but no matter how you cut it, they do not have the actual life experience, relatability, or actual encounters these group members did. I was able to get an education about bipolar without having to read about it! I was able to benefit from others and their experiences, both good and bad. Initially, I thought of it as a can of "mixed nuts", but now, looking back on it, it is more of a "treasure box" of knowledge and experiences. Every person has value. Every one of us has worth.

A fellow group member of mine once said that we do not have an illness that is better or worse than the next person, only different.

It helped me to realize that although our struggles are unique, we, individually, have something to impart, that could help someone else who may be going through something similar. Occasionally, though, there are some persons seeking help who are more needy than others and might need to be redirected to some other level of care rather than to be disruptive to the flow or progress achieved in a compatible group setting. These cases seem rare but are best handled by the Behavioral Health Professionals.

In Bipolar Group, we talk about things like our energy or mood being either high or low. We discuss whether we are tired or if we feel more like bouncing off the walls. We talk about meds, side-effects, dosages, and interactions. We discuss whether we are or are not getting sufficient exercise. We discuss our sleep levels. We talk about relationships, triggers, finances, and stressors and about the ways to navigate and tackle those challenges. We share strengths and weaknesses, as well as good or bad habits. We listen and we are heard. We laugh, and at times, we even cry. What is brought to the group stays in the group. Group members are focused on helping each other. By nature of that, the group becomes quite cohesive.

Yes, I would have to say that this Bipolar Group has been special—near and dear to my heart, in fact. It, however, is in no way more powerful than my individual therapy/counseling. I have now seen the same counselor (LPCC) who oversees the Bipolar Group, for my Individual Therapy for about eleven years. She is an excellent listener; she engages me in thought with good questions and guidance. She promotes healthy decision-making and suggests reasonable approaches to problem-solving. She hesitates and uses caution when handing out advice.

My counselor asks direct and important questions about stressors, sleep, energy, mood, medications, interpersonal relationships, and my interactions and reactions in general. The reason I mention all of this is that it might be useful in orienting some of your conversations with your doctor, therapist, provider, loved-one, etc., to include some of these topics, if they are not already being discussed. After all, "you" are a very important member of that relationship!

If you're wondering, "why would she need so many years of counseling?" my best answer would probably be "life happens, and it keeps right on happening." Life is filled with both joyous moments and stress-filled moments. I personally do not handle life's stressors very well. At one point, we had five teenagers (some with special needs) and at the same time, living with Bipolar 1, you might realize that it has been no cake walk! Counseling/therapy has been more of a blessing than a curse, and more of a necessity than a crutch. Assistance in processing life's challenges (big and small) is something most of us could benefit from, but would we be willing to admit it and ask for help?

Some people feel that recovery with Bipolar should be akin to other recoveries that one can relate to. Sort of a "just get over it", "shake it off", or an "enough already" mentality. Recovery, with bipolar, in my view, is a life-long journey. Most people must work at it daily. I have thought to liken it to oral health. A person can be proactive by brushing morning and evening, flossing, check-ups and cleanings every six months, etc., or they could opt for a lesser program. The results are generally, but not always, in the effort. I prefer to be proactive and put effort into my program and not leave my mental health to chance, especially where my family is concerned.

Life changed dramatically once the summer of 2007 ended. The kids went back to school, schedules got crazy-busy again, and although I was staying at my aunt's home, there was still much to attend to. Just attending Individualized Educational Programs (IEP) meetings alone was challenging (just in trying, not succeeding, to advocate for our kids). My brother and sister-in-law were exceedingly kind and more than generous in coming into our home half of the time. My husband was working and commuting until November 2007 when he took more than a 45% cut in pay to work in a city nearby where he would take a position with the county to be able to stay home and be fully present to us outside of his work schedule. It made a HUGE difference.

The pay-cut was an enormous change, as you can well imagine. We had to make meaningful adjustments along the way. During these years of change and challenge we were given hand-me-downs from cousins and family all around us. Generous neighbors from our community provided school supplies each fall for each of the children, all handled very thoughtfully and discreetly. Other families donated items such as used computers, video gaming consoles, etc.

An uncle would buy groceries (especially milk, as we would guzzle down about a gallon a day). He also brought Christmas gifts for each of the kids that year, something they'll always cherish. A cousin gave us winter jackets almost yearly for whichever of the kids they would fit. Another cousin would very selflessly give her gently used "brand-named" clothing to the girls to choose from. There was kindness galore!

We quickly learned that thrift store shopping was not just practical and fun, it was necessary. Sure, accepting others' generosity was humbling, but it was also a beautiful blessing.

By 2009, I was finally granted Social Security Disability Income! This involved much dedication and effort from an aunt, a special friend, and the lawyer my aunt hired. We are grateful beyond expression!

Later, around fall of 2011, while in group, I remember saying that it had been over four years since my last episode. It was the longest stretch I had gone. I was not boasting or bragging, I was simply stating it matter-of-factly, with deep gratitude.

Little did I know, that just around the corner, I would be facing another hospitalization.

Chapter 9

The Med Interaction

(Episode #7)

Several years had passed by, but certainly not without challenge! In 2012, our kids were ages seventeen, sixteen, fourteen, thirteen, and eleven. They were collectively attending five different schools. Between 2007 and 2012, our lives were filled with numerous doctor and therapy appointments for the kids (such as Art Therapy, Occupational Therapy, Psychotherapy and Family Therapy). At school, all five children had IEPs and extra-curricular schedules that also kept us busy (band, drama club, ski club, math club, Mock Trial, chess club, and tennis). The oldest went to the Teen Center, was employed, and was in Driver's Ed. Additionally, there was Church involvement (three altar servers and catechism).

I had a full-time job just getting kids from one place to another while keeping my own complicated schedule and trying, quite literally, to keep my sanity.

In September of 2009, my dad decided he would give us land on which we could build a home. We were renting my brother's home, after all. It just made the most sense when we ran the numbers, (to "cash out" our 401k, paying penalties and taxes) and build something long-term. It didn't make sense to keep dishing out thousands and thousands month after month on rent, and never have anything to show for it years down the road, especially into our older years. The stock market had taken quite a beating in 2001 and 2008, so putting our money into something solid seemed logical.

By March 23, 2010, the land was recorded in our names and soon after, two of my brothers and some other men in the community that were friends of theirs, began construction of the home I designed for our family. It was nothing fancy, just meant to house the seven of us more comfortably and more practically. It was designed to be lighter and brighter to bene-fit mood and overall well-being. A friend (who was a Drafter/ Architect) took my chicken scratch and drew up blueprints suitable for construction.

My brother was almost done with construction of our home in late 2011/early 2012, and we began preparing ourselves for the excitement (and stress) of moving. Sometime in that Fall/ Winter (2011) timeframe, I had seen my primary care doctor about a slight bit of toenail fungus. She prescribed a med for it. Long story short, the med had a synergistic (combined) effect/ interaction with a psychotropic drug I was taking. Little by little, unbeknownst to me, I fell into a mixed episode, probably due to toxicity.

My personal notes say that on November 19, 2011, I was "struggling w/moderate to severe depression." On December 31, 2011, I noted that I "felt uncomfortable, nervous, jittery" at a potluck that my brother-in-law and sister-in-law were hosting. On January 2, 2012, I remarked in my notes that I had "Facial EPS & gritting teeth." EPS stands for Extrapyramidal

Symptoms. It is a side effect of certain anti-psychotic and other drugs, causing uncontrollable movements such as tremors or muscle twitching. On January 14, 2012, I was "feeling disconnected head to body & foggy/fuzzy-headed".

Notes from the Primary Care Doctor at the Medical Center where I was being cared for:

01/19/2012

S: The patient is a 45-year-old woman who comes in today to follow-up on [Name of Psychotropic Drug] toxicity that was precipitated starting [name of anti-fungal drug prescribed]. The patient has discontinued this drug and states that she is feeling a great deal better. She is continuing the current dose of the Psychotropic drug of 10 mg daily.

The follow-up, notated just prior, was done at the prompting of my counselor who had consulted with her colleagues, a well-known psychiatrist and my primary care doctor.

The following is the discharge summary from the Regional Medical Center's Behavioral Health Unit Nine-day admission:

Date of Admission: 02/19/2012
Date of Discharge: 02/27/2012

Discharge-Transfer Documentation
Regional Medical Center
Behavioral Health Services

PSYCHIATRIC DISCHARGE SUMMARY

BRIEF SUMMARY OF PRESENT ILLNESS

This is a 45-year-old married female with history of bipolar disorder who was admitted through the emergency department on a voluntary basis. The patient presented with a chief complaint of "I was manic yesterday, the most manic I've ever been." The patient has been followed by her psychiatrist. The patient feels that her current medication regimen has been working well overall. She states that she has been overwhelmed by stress recently as she is the mother of 5 children, 2 of whom have Asperger's Syndrome. Her eldest who has Asperger's was recently hospitalized with severe dehydration and apparently had become so wrapped up in schoolwork and video games that this child was not eating and drinking properly. The patient blames herself. The patient states she almost lost them. The patient also talks about losing her pet dog recently.

HOSPITAL COURSE

The patient was admitted to inpatient psychiatry on a voluntary basis. Labs at time of admission: CMP showed a slightly elevated bilirubin of 1.7, otherwise within normal limits. CK of 714. TSH at 4.22. Acetaminophen and salicylate levels within normal limits. Urine tox was positive for tricyclics. Urine HCG was negative. CBC with diff showed elevated WBC count of 12.0 otherwise within normal limits.

The patient was continued on Abilify 10 mg at bedtime, Ativan 1mg at bedtime, Benadryl 25 mg at bedtime, Desyrel 250 mg and Synthroid 100mg. On the unit the patient did fairly well. The patient had some trouble with sleep during the initial part of hospitalization. Ativan 1mg at bedtime was added. The patient received Cipro to treat her UTI. When I met with this patient over the weekend, patient reported that she was feeling better. She was requesting for p.r.n. Abilify so she could address her racing thoughts. The patient's Abilify was continued at 10mg at bedtime and additional Abilfy 5 mg p.r.n. was added.

Patient stabilized. Today the patient denies racing thoughts. The patient reports improved sleep. The patient is confident about discharge. The patient is scheduled to see her psychiatrist on the 6th of March. The patient is given a prescription for Abilify 10 mg at bedtime. Ativan 1mg at bedtime. Benadryl 25 mg at bedtime, Desyrel 250 mg at bedtime, and Synthroid 100 mcg in the morning.

FINAL DIAGNOSES

    Axis I: Bipolar disorder mixed episode, stable

    Axis II: Deferred

    Axis III: Urinary tract infection

    Axis IV: Recent death of family pet; illness of [child]

    Axis V: Of 50

CONDITION AT THE TIME OF DISCHARGE
The patient is sleeping better. She has significant decrease in racing thoughts. The patient is not a danger to herself or others.

This episode, I was taken by ambulance, kicking and screaming (while meditating on a mantra of sorts) and cussing like a sailor. It took three or four people to get me into the ambulance and strap me down. On the ride in, I noticed a man, probably an EMT, wearing a neck-chain with a medal that popped out of his shirt.

I said something like "Are you a Catholic?", to which he said, "Yes".

I then said something like, "I normally never ever cuss", to which he replied, "Well you sure used up more than your share today!"

When I arrived at the hospital, I was taken to the ER. They put me in a room, not a padded room, but a quiet room. I was not very quiet. In fact, for some reason, I became exceedingly loud, in an almost erotic manner. I have learned the hard way that you cannot choose your crazy; that is for sure!

My poor husband was finally able to come to the hospital and tells me now that he could hear some wild person screaming, and that as they directed him to me, the sound got louder. He greeted somebody he recognized from his work, and then continued in the direction of the sound. The sounds were, in fact, coming from me, from the nearby room I had been put in. I can only imagine how embarrassed he must have been, and still must be, to this very day. I have put him through so much. All I can do is say that I am sorry and try my best to prioritize wellness and equilibrium.

I was strapped to the bed and had been heavily sedated on separate occasions while awaiting news of a psych consult and/or availability of a bed in Behavioral Health. As briefly as I can explain, it felt like a crucifixion-like scenario (there's the religiosity). I came in and out of consciousness with my arms outstretched upward against the rails and therefore slightly numb but tingling with pain. It made me think, ever so minutely, of the death of Christ, but in a psychotic manner.

I entered a Mental Health Hospital, now for the seventh time. I haven't mentioned this before, but each mental health hospitalization requires a full body examination. They take note of each scar, scratch, bump, and bruise. This is done for documentation, but being subjected to this is dehumanizing, nonetheless.

I stayed for nine days to get stabilized and was released with the belief (*their* belief) that I would be fine. I, personally, had my doubts, as with most of the discharges.

Chapter 10

Shopped Until I Dropped

(Episode #8)

Somehow, from about late-February (previous discharge) up through about mid-May 2012 (this next episode), I spent about $14,000 on trivial, frivolous, ridiculous and impulsive purchases. To give you a rough idea of the madness, below is a list of purchases made in that timeframe as an example of those hypo-manic/manic events.

1. ~$1000 spent all at once at a large Drugstore chain nearby
2. ~$1500 spent in about 2 visits to a big box General Merchandise store
3. ~$1500 spent all at once at a big box Club/Warehouse store
4. ~$3000 spent all in one trip at a big box Hardware Store
5. $2450 on the purchase of a 1996 Honda Civic
6. $2450 on a 1977 Toyota Dolphin (Recreational Vehicle)
7. ~$700 on tires for the RV
8. ~$1500 on items at a silent auction

Some of the items could be returned, others could not. I was probably able to return about $1000 to $1500 in merchandise once the dust settled. The seriousness of this manic episode had me essentially unaccounted for at one point, for about two days, at the near climax of it all. I opened two to three credit card accounts and was driving everyone in my path crazy.

Regarding the purchase of the RV, during the time when I was unaccounted for, I met a man at a car wash, who was washing his RV. I guess I must have asked him if he would sell his RV, because he didn't have a 'for sale' sign on it. Remember that it seemed as if I had rose colored glasses on, and everything seemed better than it was. The RV was light blue and white, and reminded me of the Blessed Virgin Mary.

It had sheepskin seat covers and satellite radio, which all seemed very upscale to me. Upon discussing the matter, we arrived at a sales price of $2,450. As things unfolded, I came to realize that he was actually living in the RV, and without it would have been completely homeless. With selling the RV, he would then be able to put money down on an apartment. We needed to get paperwork from MVD, and I would need to go to the bank, so I got a motel for the night. Realizing that he was essentially without facilities, I allowed him to take a shower at the motel while I waited outside.

The reason I'm sharing this with you is that looking back on it, I now realize what a danger I put myself in. An instance like this could have easily led to a bad outcome. Anyone observing from the outside would have probably considered it a marital indiscretion. Thankfully, nothing happened, and he went on his way. We met the next day and took care of the transaction.

Another reason I chose to write this is because oftentimes persons with bipolar disorder can be subject to hypersexual behaviors during an episode, and even in general. So, one would want to be incredibly careful regarding their decisions and their actions. It is not unheard of for this illness to cause behaviors that can lead to divorce and/or broken relationships.

Regarding item number eight above, my husband, daughter, and I attended a Japanese cultural convention, whereby I proceeded to place bids on most of the items up for auction. It was quite a spectacle in that no sooner would I sign my name for an item than my husband would quickly follow to scratch my name off in hopes that he could thwart my manic spending spree. I can honestly say my self-awareness was outrageously poor, and I was absolutely not acting out intentionally. The items they were unable to rescue me from had to be purchased and could not be returned. Unfortunately, each manic/hypomanic episode went hand-in-hand with a terrific amount of spending.

I must have appeared, at least, to be keeping it somewhat together. I was keeping some, if not most, of my appointments for therapy, psychiatry, etc. I was coming and going and functioning relatively well during most of that time, but hospitalization was soon my reality.

By May, I was in the regretful, "aware of my actions" phase, and was quite depressed. I was having mild to moderate bouts with suicidality. One temptation or struggle was with the thought that I would throw a blow-dryer in the tub with me. Another still was jumping off a bridge. Several other thoughts and ideas came in waves, some stronger than others. Fortunately, I was able to get help in a timely manner. I had an appointment with my psychiatrist, and she suggested that I go to the emergency room. I called my husband to come take me.

When I arrived at the behavioral health unit, I was once again subjected to the routine body search. This already-difficult experience was made worse when I realized that the search would be performed by a staff member who had made a casual threat to me during my prior hospitalization. I was already in a bad space due to my depression, and emotionally challenged with the thought that this person could possibly manipulate my records/treatment.

I believed this hospitalization would end with me being permanently institutionalized. It was documented that I said, "It's over for me, I can feel it this time.". I was convinced this was the last straw. I was moderately to severely depressed and was feeling quite agonized about what might be next. From a deep dark place, it is hard to visualize anything lovely. Your mind essentially robs you of that.

Discharge Summary from the Regional Medical Center's Behavioral Health Unit seven-day admission:

Date of Admission: 05/17/2012

Date of Discharge: 05/23/2012

Discharge-Transfer Documentation
Regional Medical Center
Behavioral Health Services

HISTORY OF PRESENT ILLNESS
This is a 45-year-old married female, mother of 5 with history of bipolar disorder followed by (name of psychiatrist) at

(specific name of center). The patient is admitted through the emergency room after reporting suicidal ideation. The patient presented with a chief complaint of "I am suffering from a post hypomanic state." The patient states that she has been compliant with her treatment. The patient was in a hypomanic state in February and during that phase the patient spent a lot of money. The patient states that she spent about $12,000 in buying an RV which is not in very good shape. The patient also bought lots of unwanted things from (name of pharmacy) and from (name of Big Box Hardware Store) which she has returned some of it.

The patient now feels very inadequate, worthless and has had suicidal thoughts for the last 2 weeks. The patient states that she has had prescriptions for several different medicines that she has access to and had thoughts of overdosing on these medicines. The patient saw (name of psychiatrist) yesterday who referred her to the emergency room. During this interview, the patient also talked about her new house which she herself designed. The patient states that there is not enough room to accommodate all her belongings and there are a lot of boxes in her garage. The patient reported feeling hopeless, helpless. The patient complained of poor sleep, fair appetite, steady weight. The patient denies racing thoughts. The patient denies symptoms of psychosis. There are no substance abuse issues.

HOSPITAL COURSE
The patient was admitted to impatient psychiatry on a voluntary basis. Labs at the time of admission showed a CMP within normal limits. TSH is at 0.4. Urine tox was negative. Urine pregnancy was negative. CBC with diff showed a slightly elevated WBC of 11.2, otherwise within normal limits. UA was within normal limits. The patient was continued on Abilify 30 mg nightly and Synthroid 125 mcg in the morning with Trazodone 200 mg at bedtime.

Patient was started on Lithium with the intentions to help this patient with mood stability and suicidality. Risks and benefits were discussed. The patient was started on Lithium Carbonate 300 mg 3 times a day. The patient tolerated the medicine well, salicylate level on the 22nd was at 0.6. The patient reports some improvement in mood. The patient now is denying suicidality. A family meeting was done with patient's husband, various/different interventions were discussed. Need for this patient to not have access to the family savings and having access to limited amount of money has been discussed. Need for possibly engaging in DBT (Dialectical Behavioral Therapy) was discussed. The patient's husband is supportive of this patient. The patient would like to switch to Tegretol if she does not feel like Lithium is working. Today the patient reports improvement in mood and is denying suicidality. The patient is worried about her children. The plan is for the patient to go live with her sister-in-law for a short period of time. The patient will follow up with (name of psychiatrist) tomorrow on 5/24/2012. The patient is to continue Abilify 30 mg at bedtime, Trazodone 200 mg at bedtime, Lithobid 300 mg 3 times a day and Synthroid 125 mcg in the morning. The patient has enough supply of her medicines. The only prescription the patient was discharged on is Lithobid 300 mg 3 times a day. The patient received a prescription for 3 weeks

FINAL DIAGNOSES
Axis I: Bipolar affective disorder, type 1, depressed.
Axis II: Deferred.
Axis III: History of Hypothyroidism.
Axis IV: Chronic illness, financial issues.
Axis V: 50.

PLAN

At the time of discharge, risk assessment has been done. Patient's risk for suicide at this time is low.

Upon discharge, I was considered as not being a danger to myself or others, and as always, I followed up with all scheduled appointments, took my meds as adjusted by the hospital psychiatrist, and tried to pick up the pieces once more.

As of this writing, it has been ten years after the eighth episode. I still see a therapist once a week, see a psychiatrist about every six to eight weeks, take my meds as advised, attend Bipolar Group weekly, and outside of the pandemic, still sought respite at my aunt's house about twice monthly. I still take medication daily, and it is still a bit of a pharmaceutical cocktail. No surprise there.

I recognize that somehow along the way, I have failed to mention a couple of key things along my route. One thing was that upon each hospitalization, my sister-in-law provided me with a rosary to pray. It helped with the inevitable pacing by giving my hands and mind something to do other than focus on my worries, fears, and doubts. Rather, I would walk and pray. To this day, I love to walk and pray. They say, "**take care of body, soul and mind.**" Personally, I feel that if you take care of the first two, you in turn take care of the latter.

Another key thing was what I often did *between* hospitalizations in keeping with wellness. I worked out with either my cousin or my "sos" (sister-oh-sister). Either way, we found ourselves walking and laughing (literally hunched over laughing) and carrying on! I did not have sisters growing up, so I now cling to the women in my life like Velcro.

As of May 13th of 2022, it's been 21 years into this diagnosis of Bipolar 1. It has been nearly ten years without an episode! In honor of those milestones, I celebrate! I survived! I am eternally grateful that I did.

During a proofreading session with my "sos" that was focused on run-on sentences, she shared with me a beautiful quote that nearly made me cry. It sums up quite well what this book really is all about:

"ONE DAY YOU WILL TELL YOUR STORY OF HOW YOU OVERCAME WHAT YOU WENT THROUGH, AND IT WILL BE SOMEONE ELSE'S SURVIVAL GUIDE." - BRENÉ BROWN

Trust me, my life has been no picnic. With medicine, therapy, proper self-care, a good attitude, plenty of support (and for me, with trust and dependence on God), it has been a lot more stable. I have become more peaceful, and I am much happier. The beauty of this ride now, is that I can liken it to more of a *pleasure ride*. It has fewer big ups and downs, and now has more gentle, manageable turns.

That pretty much wraps up the autobiographical component of this written work. I feel that in completing this book I honor my journey, and that by writing about my experiences and sharing them with others, it makes the "*struggle*" all worthwhile.

Chapter 11

Insights, Tips & Strategies

That concludes the eight episodes as best I can remember each. The years since have not been easy. They rarely are. For the most part, however, they have been relatively smooth overall. Thankfully, I have not been hospitalized (knock on wood) and have not suffered any serious hypomania, mania, or depression.

For those of you who read the entire account, thank you for sticking with me. I hope that at least something I shared can be useful.

As was customary in treating Bipolar in 2001, upon each discharge from the Mental Hospital, I was given appointments for counseling and psychiatry. Unfortunately, not enough emphasis was placed on education, accountability, understanding and follow-up. As I have said previously, knowledge is power. I strongly suggest that you, the reader, research and do your homework, so that you are as proactive in dealing with your situation as possible.

It is probably not necessary to understand every aspect of one's treatment goals in detail, although it certainly does not hurt. It most definitely helps to have at least a basic understanding. I entered my situation with blinders on, something I absolutely do not recommend. At that time, search engines were in their infancy, and people were much less informed, or should I say, much less likely to pursue getting informed.

Initially, it was hard to wrap my head around the idea of taking medicine at all. For me, not only was I ignorant as to how important daily doses were, but I was ignorant of the importance of keeping meds refilled, the necessity of making and keeping regular appointments with my doctor, and the need for regular therapy.

My world was busy enough already, and it was hard to justify time for anything more. I learned over time, and unfortunately, the hard way, that these meds, these appointments, the therapy, the doctor visits, the pharmacy refills, etc., were all designed to be done for my benefit. They were necessary components of my follow-up care and were not meant to be optional.

Whether a person chooses to medicate, self-medicate, or not medicate is a personal choice. Each person must make an honest personal assessment of their own. Some people may have fewer responsibilities and can risk that their mood, energy, and activity will be unpredictable. One will learn over a period of time how their life is negatively impacted by poor sleep, fluctuations in overall behavioral health, and the positive or negative interactions that they might have with family, friends, authority, co-workers, etc.

Honestly, to this very day, I do not enjoy taking meds; in fact, I highly dislike it. Filling a medicine tray each week, keeping track of dosages, refills, trips to the pharmacy, expiration dates, etc. is not a fun way to spend your time. What I can say is that for me, the price to pay is way larger without meds on-board. My life, and the impact on my family, are way too important to risk not taking meds.

So anyhow, below is a list of *thoughts and opinions* you could refer to in terms of seeking and/or maintaining wellness while living with Bipolar. These are provided based on approaches I have opted for, or that I have known of others to choose, that have proven to be beneficial to quality of life or one's general well-being (they are numbered fairly randomly, so try not to focus on any specific order of importance):

1. Psychiatry:

Psychiatrists prescribe the medicine for their patient and educate them regarding desired effects, side-effects, and drug interactions which can be quite useful during startup of a med, or during med changes. Initially, it is likely that you will need to see your psychiatrist once, maybe even twice a week. Further down the road, that may change to twice a month, then once a month, depending on how you stabilize and if there are complications with regulating you on meds. Currently, I see my psychiatrist about every six to eight weeks to check in and to have her write scripts for those without refills, or those coming up before our next visit. Regular check-ins with your psychiatrist are beneficial to help them evaluate how you are doing overall in terms of your mental health.

2. Medication:

For those opting to use meds, it is probable that your doctor may prescribe a combination of some or all of the following: a good mood stabilizer, an anti-depressant, an anti-psychotic, and a sleep med. Some require bloodwork to determine whether the med is in a therapeutic range or if it reaches a level of toxicity. At first, doing all these things is foreign (like filling prescriptions, filling pill boxes/trays, and doing lab work) but after some time it just seems like part of your day. I may not like it, but it is necessary. Sometimes, it is just easier to accept things in life and not complain about them. At any given time, I might have ten to fifteen pills in my tray at bedtime. For me, it is a no-brainer; I could not even begin to imagine life now, without meds.

3. Therapy/Counseling:

Finding a good therapist is key to helping reduce stress-ors and having a means with which to decompress. Therapy/ Counseling is valuable to provide healthy guidance in handling life's stressors. Something worth mentioning is that you will probably be referred to someone immediately after a hospitali-zation. This does not mean that it will be a good match for you or that you will connect on any level. I would say that two to four sessions should be sufficient in determining whether that relationship works for you. Do not be afraid to look elsewhere in hope of a better fit. It is worth re-hashing your story, even a few times, in order to get a good connection. There could be any number of reasons why you would choose to find some-one new, but your reasons are valid to you and are not worth ignoring.

4. Sleep:

Likely one of the most important items in this list, in my opinion, is getting good regular sleep (quality and quantity), so much so, that it is worth starting a habit of setting an alarm for the time you take your medicine each evening, then devoting yourself to going straight to bed. Eliminate sights and sounds of anything not conducive to sleep, such as your cell phone, TV, computer, and the like. Work to develop a habit of setting a wake alarm for a timeframe that allows for six to twelve hours of sleep, eight probably being a good goal.

I have been through stages of depression whereby I got twelve or more hours easily, and naps. You simply must work within the parameters that you are dealing with and ease toward a goal little by little. When manic, I have gone without sleep for days. The idea is to move toward stability using all your resources, and once regulated, work hard to try to stay there. I treat sleep like anything I value highly because it has proven to be a critical ingredient to balanced mental health.

5. Med Trials/Changes:

At first, I tried several medications that either proved to be ineffective or proved to have adverse side-effects and/or reactions. Trial and error quickly became part of my life, as well as additional episodes and hospitalizations. This is not to say that anything I have to say will offer you a short-cut to this trial-and-error process, but hopefully just knowing that this can be part of the process, and even just being informed that you may have to endure this, should help. Perseverance and patience are half the battle, and it is one worth fighting. It is my experience that a person must be careful when making changes to medication due to allergic reactions or medication interactions, even with over-the-counter medications and supplements. Proceed with caution! Using a medication-interaction app is very helpful.

6. Primary Care Doctor:

Keeping track of and staying on top of physical health issues are especially important. There may be underlying health issues such as diabetes, thyroid issues, kidney and liver monitoring, etc. that are good for you to keep up to speed on. If you are fortunate, you can have most, if not all, of your providers come from one medical group, providing it has a Behavioral Health Department. This can make it easier to coordinate care so that providers/colleagues can communicate more readily on your behalf. For example, if your energy is low, it might be affected by a separate health issue and may not require a med adjustment from the "Bipolar Department". One may be deficient in B-vitamins or have a thyroid issue that a primary care provider can attend to.

7. Bipolar Support:

NAMI (National Alliance for the Mentally Ill) provides support for self, family and friends. Contact info: nami.org, and the NAMI Help Line 1-800-950-NAMI (6264).

8. Bipolar Group:

I highly recommend attending a Bipolar Group at least three or four times to get a semi-decent feel for it. A visit or two is not enough, in my opinion, to recognize its value. That would be like taking only one hour in Yellowstone or at a major theme park. Within the text of this book, I give my reasons for learning to appreciate Bipolar Group, but it is not a *necessary* component. That said, I would highly recommend it.

9. Warning Signs:

It is helpful to get acquainted with the early signs of depression and mania, and to consider how they apply to you, your body, and your tendencies. How do you feel? What are you experiencing early on? What are your thoughts? Make a mental or written list specific to you and keep the list handy for reference. Consider sharing this information (written and/or verbal) with someone you are close to and who you trust.

10. Hypomania & Mania:

Personally, I find it hard to distinguish the marker from one to the other; it seemingly happens so fast. Self-monitoring and frequent check-ins are a must. Typically, for me, I feel extremely caffeinated and jittery or speedy when hypomanic. Shopping is highly discouraged, especially for big-ticket items, during the hypomanic thru mania timeframe. If I notice I am feeling even slightly revved or a bit too happy or energetic, or sleep-deprived, I generally take something within my arsenal of supplements or as-needed prescription meds to calm/slow me down or to get some sleep. This often can prevent one from rocketing into full-blown mania.

It is different for everybody, but for me, mania means it is time to go to the hospital. This is for my own and others' safety from financial, verbal and/or psychological harm. In mania, I am hardly myself, and have been known to cause confusion, stress, concern, hurt, and pain, all at the price of becoming irregular.

11. Depression:

Dealing with Depression can be a huge struggle. In addition to self-monitoring and using your "Go-To" lists and/or known resources, I suggest you try to take in some light, try to stretch, try to move your body even if just a bit. Let in some fresh air. Attempt to make a list of things you think you can still do (especially those things that help you feel better), based on how you are feeling. Work on doing the things on your list little by little. It is important to reach out to someone you trust to help you pull out of this, especially, if the Depression advances toward serious or severe.

If suicidal thoughts ever do crop up, refer to #19. However, if you start to have suicidal ideation (more than having suicidal thoughts alone), and you are making plans, call 911 immediately.

12. Overcoming Stigma:

Mental illness comes with a heaping serving of stigma. What is the image you get when you first hear "mentally ill person"? If we are honest, most of us probably picture a street person or a person behaving outrageously, right? Sometimes we judge too easily; we are all probably guilty of it to one degree or another, but as best we are able, we should try to have compassion for those who suffer from a mental illness. None of us can say with absolute certainty that it will never happen to someone we love or know, much less ourselves. It's healthy to consider how we would feel and how we might handle ourselves in someone else' shoes.

The best advice I can give is "Live well and do your best not to add to the stigma." Try your level best to get and stay stable and try to maintain an attitude and posture of being healthy and happy despite the disorder. It is hard enough to maintain one's own peace, let alone deal with the negativity and bad rap associated with the stigma of persons with mental illness, or more specifically, bipolar disorder. **You MUST NOT allow this illness to define who you are.**

13. Exercise:

Exercise is a wonderful investment in your mental health & wellness. Regardless of what level you can participate (depending on your health limitations), if you are able to move, then move. Fast or slow, big movements or small movements, with or without weights, and with or without the help of machines and or assistance. Move your body, stretch your body, and allow yourself to derive the benefits of increased health, improved sleep, and likely improved mood.

14. Quiet Time:

A quote by William Penn: **"True silence is the rest of the mind, and is to the spirit what sleep is to the body, nourishment and refreshment."** In this busy day and age, it is hard to "take space", or find or create quiet moments, but it is possible. A person simply needs to carve out time for it, even set an alarm at a desirable part of each day. Maybe take a minute or two initially, then slowly increase the time you spend, whether in silence, in meditation of some sort, or in prayer. Just quieting the mind, quite simply, is the goal. Some people use candles, others calming sounds of nature or soft music. Any way you choose. Increase the time according to your life. A goal might be 10 minutes that you give yourself. Personally, I have slowly increased my quiet time, prayer, and devotion to roughly about an hour, and sometimes more, each day.

15. Mood & Energy:

Regulating mood & energy is hard work for most of us with bipolar. It involves exercise, eating healthy well- balanced meals, proper sleep, hygiene, self-monitoring, repeat. This is true for someone who is stable. From the standpoint of someone who is severely unstable or episodic, this would be secondary to getting regulated. This could mean a visit to the ER to have a psychiatric evaluation performed for the possibility of a Behavior Health hospitalization.

16. Triggers:

What can cause your mood to lift or lower suddenly? What can set you off in either direction? Familiarize yourself with these triggers (persons, places and things, situations, etc.) and consider their cause. Then, avoid or minimize these whenever and wherever you can to lessen impact/symptoms.

17. Stress:

Reduce stress with whatever in the following list works for you: Talk therapy, meditation, prayer, exercise, music, sunshine, herbal tea, aromatherapy, laughter, bubble bath, candles, quiet time, a massage, nature, loving on pets, opening the window and doors, or anything healthy and pleasurable. Work to reduce stress daily, if not hourly.

18. Anxiety:

You can take calming prescription meds or supplements. You can use weighted blankets, aromatherapy and/or drink herbal tea. A person can distract themselves with a calm or funny movie or television show, or as with most stressful situations, you can talk to a trusted friend or therapist. Hug someone or something.

19. Suicidal Thoughts:

Call the National Suicide Prevention Lifeline at 1-800-273-TALK (8255), and/or seek immediate professional help, or go to the Emergency Room. Please do everything you can possibly do or think of to stay alive. There is only one, wonderful, precious you! Please get help! **However, if you start to have suicidal ideation (more than having suicidal thoughts alone), where you are making plans, call 911 immediately.**

20. Employer Disclosure:

This is an extremely difficult/sensitive consideration. A well-thought-out approach is a must; err on the side of caution. This is due largely in part to stigma. Disclosure about your illness to an employer can often interfere with being considered for a promotion, job loss, not being selected for a leadership role or a position of trust, or any other form of discrimination. Proceed with caution. Many people feel a sense of relief and freedom in finally divulging this information to others, so it seems that it might also make sense to disclose at work. Evaluate carefully. The bigger/better the job, perhaps, the greater one's potential for risk/loss.

21. Follow-up:

Whether a diagnosis is made on an in-patient or out-patient basis, proper follow-up is vital, even if only to get a second opinion. Following through with appointments, medications, etc. is highly recommended. Researching your diagnosis and evaluating your options is worthy of careful consideration but remember that time is of the essence in getting the care you might need.

22. Medical Records:

I cannot emphasize enough that you request and pay for your medical records from a mental health hospital and/or behavioral health care organization. Do this in as timely a fashion as possible after treatment has been completed. Trust me on this. The education, hindsight and objectivity alone is extremely valuable.

23. Support:

Support is a key element in one's ability to handle this difficult illness. It is easy to alienate those who try to help us, especially if we are not regulated. It is not easy to accept others' help. In fact, it is quite difficult. I was told later that I was uneasy in accepting people's help, and that I was down-right ugly in the way I treated some people during certain episodes. I deeply regret any injury I may have caused anyone. I would advise that you keep this in mind as you work to-wards becoming stable. I realize that not everyone has an ideal support system. That is where choosing a therapist and/or a support group can be vital.

24. Denial & Acceptance:

It took several episodes for me to get past denial. I did not have a good handle on what I was dealing with or what to expect. Change does not come easily to most folks; I was no exception. Acceptance of this diagnosis is a process. It hap-pened for me over a long period of time. Just recently, I was able to finally relate to a situation my mother was involved in with one of her episodes. I could not accept or come to grips with her behavior, until I experienced similar behavior during one of my own episodes.

Personally, I think that the assessment and evaluation tools used to diagnose bipolar, should at least be discussed with the patient. Education, accountability and follow-thru are all helpful in coming out of denial and into acceptance.

Chapter 12

So Far, So Good!

I have five big reasons for this tiny chapter.

First, it would help to mention that although I would love to make a promise, I could never promise that I will not have any additional episodes in the future. That is just something, by the nature of this beast, I cannot guarantee. I will, however, promise to work ridiculously hard to stay well. I liken my attitude to that of a person in the movie "Magnificent Seven" where the actor Chris Pratt tells of a fella who fell off a five-story building. Passing each story on the way down, people heard the fella say, "So far, so good!". In other words, I want to try to keep a good attitude regardless of how long or how short a time I have on this earth. The way I see it, things could be better, BUT, they could also be WORSE. I *strive* to be content and happy with what I have.

I have an aunt who has been battling cancer for a long time (since 2008); she has set the bar for me as a model for being amazingly strong, and for having an excellent attitude.

Second, I *hope* that somehow this book "scratched the surface," so to speak, at least *slightly*! My goal was to share and remember as honestly as I could, each episode. Another goal was to offer strategies that might be enough to cause a person to seek diagnosis and treatment, and to encourage full engagement in one's own treatment plan. I hope I have met those goals well enough, even if only for one other person!

Third, is to be sure to convey that I have severe feelings of indebtedness to family, friends and neighbors for all that must have happened, and all that was involved in helping us. This indebtedness remains to this day. I could never do anything to repay any one person, much less repay ALL the people who have helped us in some shape or form. It is eight episodes later, and we are still healing from each one. I cannot stress enough as to how I know in my heart, that I could never properly thank everyone individually, but I thought that in writing this book, it would also show my gratitude. I am left simply to say, "Thank You!! I am truly appreciative of all that has been done on my behalf and to make "*my struggle to be well*" a whole lot easier.

Fourth, is to say that just about any other man would have left me. I love my husband so much for standing by me through all of this. He has been so incredible, not just in that one way, but in so many countless ways! May God always bless you, my Teddy Bear. I love you!

Fifth, in addressing readers who are seeking help for themselves, or for a loved one, there are many choices, and many paths one could follow. What worked for me may not work for you. Please keep searching, and you will come up with what works best for you in your own situation. Alas, I say thank you for reading, best wishes, stay safe (this book was completed during the Coronavirus Pandemic) and be well.

Acknowledgments

I wish to thank:

God, for His love, patience, guidance, and endless mercy,
my very dedicated and loving husband for his
commitment, loyalty, and friendship,
our five children, for their resilience, love, compassion,
and fortitude,
our immediate & extended family, friends, and
neighbors, for all their help and support,
an extraordinary counselor, for her expertise, dedication
and tireless care,
all our providers, for their efforts in assisting our family
to maintain balance over the years,
and all the helping and praying hands that gave us
support, there are just too many to mention.

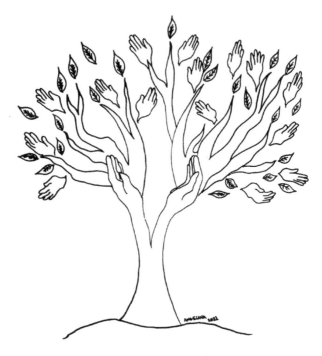

Gratitude Tree
Angelina Vigil

Regarding this book, I am especially thankful for:
those persons who helped encourage, read, proofread,
critique, and edit prior to publishing,
Justine Manzano, for her editing expertise and
encouragements,
Rachel, for her assistance with edits, the beautiful cover
art, website design, and misc. time,
Theresa, for formatting the book and for overall
logistical and promotional support,
James, for fundraising and promotional efforts,
Angelina, for the Gratitude Tree drawing above,
Jamie Mariscal for graphic design support.

Meet the Author

Aurelia is a wife of 28 years and a mother to five adult children. She received her Associates degree in Electronics Technology in 1988, and worked in that field until 1996, when she decided to be a stay-at-home mom. She and her husband volunteer for various ministries, and at church whenever possible.

She is passionate about sharing her experience living with bipolar disorder, and feels that her faith and spirituality have contributed greatly to the wellness plan that she dedicates herself to. She recognizes that each person's journey is unique, and hopes that they can also make peace with their illness.

CPSIA information can be obtained
at www.ICGtesting.com
Printed in the USA
JSHW030903300123
36876JS00004B/306